Practice Nurse

About the Editor

Tina Bishop has worked as a Practice Nurse since the mid-1980s and undertakes regular clinical practice. Her clinical interest includes women's health and wound care. Tina has a very keen interest in role development and has developed and established many programmes to support nurses working in general practice, including the Practice Nurse Apprenticeship Scheme in association with Primary Care Education in South Essex. Tina has recently developed and leads the Non-Medical Prescribing Programme. Her current role also includes working with trusts and service providers in developing new programmes to support practice. She is a member of the editorial board of the *Practice Nurse* journal and is also a member of the RCN Committee of the Practice Nurse Forum.

For Elsevier:

Associate Editor: Mairi McCubbin
Project Manager: Jess Thompson
Cover Design: Kneath Associates
Typesetting and Production: Helius

Advanced Practice Nurse

Edited by

Tina Bishop BSc(Hons) MA DipN PGCE RGN

Practice Nurse and Senior Lecturer, Community Nursing,
Anglia Ruskin University, Chelmsford, UK

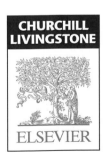

CHURCHILL
LIVINGSTONE

ELSEVIER

Edinburgh   London   New York   Oxford   Philadelphia   St Louis   Sydney   Toronto   2007

CHURCHILL
LIVINGSTONE
ELSEVIER

An imprint of Elsevier Limited

First published 2007

ISBN-10: 0 443 10263 5
ISBN-13: 978 0 443 10263 9

British Library Cataloguing in Publication Data
A catalogue record for this book is available from the British Library

Library of Congress Cataloging in Publication Data
A catalog record for this book is available from the Library of Congress

Notice
Knowledge and best practice in this field are constantly changing. As new research and experience broaden our knowledge, changes in practice, treatment and drug therapy may become necessary or appropriate. Readers are advised to check the most current information provided (i) on procedures featured or (ii) by the manufacturer of each product to be administered, to verify the recommended dose or formula, the method and duration of administration, and contraindications. It is the responsibility of the practitioner, relying on their own experience and knowledge of the patient, to make diagnoses, to determine dosages and the best treatment for each individual patient, and to take all appropriate safety precautions. To the fullest extent of the law, neither the Publisher nor the Editor assumes any liability for any injury and/or damage to persons or property arising out or related to any use of the material contained in this book.

The Publisher

 your source for books,
journals and multimedia
in the health sciences
www.elsevierhealth.com

The
publisher's
policy is to use
**paper manufactured
from sustainable forests**

Printed in Spain

Contents

Contributors

Tina Bishop BSc(Hons) MA DipN PGCE RGN
Practice Nurse and Senior Lecturer, Anglia
Ruskin University, Chelmsford

Patricia Brown BSc(Hons) MSc RNT FETC
DipN(Lond) RGN MITLHE
Senior Lecturer, Anglia Ruskin University,
Chelmsford

Alyson Buck BSc(Hons) MA RMN RGN SCM
Senior Lecturer Mental Health, Anglia Ruskin
University, Chelmsford

Liz Fairclough
Health Services Manager, Learning and
Information Services, London South Bank
University, London

Debbie Fisher
Information Adviser (Health), Learning and
Information Services, London South Bank
University, London

Gwen Hall BSc(Hons) RMN RGN
Diabetic Nurse Specialist and Practice Nurse
Trainer, Guildford and Waverley PCT

Graham Harris MA BEd(Hons) DipN(Lond)
CertCouns RGN RNT
Senior Lecturer, Anglia Ruskin University,
Chelmsford

Angie Heini BSc(Hons) RGN
Specialist Practice Nurse and Practice Nurse
Trainer, Harlow

Sarah Kraszewski BEd PGDip RGN
Practice Nurse, Family Planning Trainer and
Senior Lecturer, Anglia Ruskin University,
Chelmsford

Maurice Wakeham
Academic Liaison Librarian, Health and Social
Care, Anglia Ruskin University, Chelmsford

Preface

Nurses are at the forefront of providing a range of services for patients. This book presents a series of topics for primary care nurses working in advancing roles and nurse-led services.

Written by nurses actively involved in providing clinical care for patients with a strong emphasis on patient care, each chapter begins with an introduction to the topic. Learning is integral to the entire text and readers are invited to relate learning to their own practice through a series of activities. Learning points are summarised and evaluation activities are suggested. Each chapter is fully referenced with further information of web-based resources when appropriate.

Tina Bishop

Acknowledgements

Grateful thanks go to all those nurses who have taken the time to contribute to this book, without whose skills and knowledge this book would never have been possible.

Section 1

Management of long-term illness

SECTION CONTENTS

Chapter 1

ASTHMA
Prevention and detection

Angie Heini

CHAPTER CONTENTS

LEARNING OBJECTIVES

After reading this chapter you will be able to:

- describe the signs and symptoms that may indicate a diagnosis of asthma
- know the objective measurements necessary to make a diagnosis of asthma
- discuss indications for referral to a specialist or for further investigations
- be aware of primary and secondary interventions for the prevention of asthma

The advent in 1990 of health-promotion clinics in general practice revolutionised the management of asthma in primary care. More recently, the *British Guideline on the Management of Asthma* and the new GMS contract have prompted an increase in the number of nurse-run asthma clinics offering comprehensive programmes of care.[1, 2]

ACTIVITY

Familiarise yourself with the *British Guideline on the Management of Asthma* and Section 8 (pp. 60–66) of the GMS contract.

Review the records of ten asthma patients, and count how many times they were seen with respiratory problems before a diagnosis of asthma was made.

Practice nurses have a key role in the diagnosis and management of asthma, and also in helping their practice achieve the clinical indicators for the new contract.

EPIDEMIOLOGY

An estimated 5.1 million people in England are being treated for asthma, at an annual cost to the NHS of around £850 million. However, it is estimated that 8 million people in the UK – around one in seven of the population – have been diagnosed with asthma at some stage in their lives.[3] An average GP sees 85 people with asthma each year, each of these consulting about three times.[4] A recent survey by the Global Initiative for Asthma (GINA) found that children in the UK have more asthma symptoms than children anywhere else in the world, with the prevalence of severe wheeze being particularly high in those aged 13–14 years.[5]

Although asthma responds well to appropriate management the condition is often poorly controlled. Many patients experience symptoms that might be relieved if treatment was reviewed and made more appropriate. More than 1,500 people still die of the condition each year in the UK and many of those deaths are potentially avoidable.[6] Asthma causes considerable physical and psychological morbidity in terms of:

- anxiety and social stigma
- impact on schooling, work and social activities
- restricted growth in some children.[1]

The cause of asthma is not completely understood, although it has long been established that its aetiology has a strong genetic component.[7] As this component has not changed, the increase in the prevalence of asthma over the past 25 years could be attributable to environmental factors. These may include changes in diet, increased use of central heating and soft furnishings, and maternal smoking. There is also wide geographical variation in the prevalence of the condition,

which is more common in urban than rural communities. Visits to the GP because of asthma are particularly frequent among people from disadvantaged social groups and certain ethnic and minority groups.[8]

DEFINITION

There is no agreed gold-standard definition of asthma. An International Consensus Report describes it as:

a chronic inflammatory disorder of the airways ... in susceptible individuals, inflammatory symptoms are usually associated with widespread but variable airflow obstruction and an increase in airway response to a variety of stimuli. Obstruction is often reversible, either spontaneously or with treatment.[9]

The BTS/SIGN guideline describes asthma as a disorder characterised by inflammation and narrowing of the airways, which can produce symptoms of wheezing, cough, chest tightness and breathlessness.[1] However, none of these symptoms is specific for asthma. The hallmark of asthma symptoms is that they tend to be:

- variable
- intermittent
- worse at night
- provoked by triggers (e.g. exercise).

DIAGNOSIS

It can be difficult to diagnose asthma, as there is no confirmatory diagnostic blood test or radiographic or histopathological investigation. However, a nurse should be suspicious whenever a patient presents with cough, wheeze, shortness of breath or chest tightness. In addition, it is important to remember that asthma symptoms are not present all of the time and therefore may be absent when the patient attends the surgery.[10]

Reversibility of airflow obstruction can be quickly tested when the patient presents, unless they are asymptomatic at the time; in that event, they can be given a peak expiratory flow (PEF) diary card to complete at home, to check for diurnal variation.

The diagnosis of asthma has to be a clinical one, and should be made with the help of the evidence-based BTS/SIGN guideline, which was developed to help practitioners decide on the most appropriate care for people with the condition (Boxes 1.1 to 1.3).[1]

Most trained asthma nurses are experienced in measuring PEF and performing spirometry, but it is worth investigating whether GP colleagues in the practice are equally competent. It may be more appropriate to train healthcare assistants to carry out these tasks, leaving the GP and nurse with more time for chronic disease management.

DIAGNOSIS IN YOUNG CHILDREN

In children under 8 years of age it can be difficult to differentiate wheezing attacks caused by asthma from those associated with other conditions such as viral infections. They cannot reliably perform PEF measurements, although many children aged 6 years and over will be able to cooperate with PEF measurements or spirometry. Equally, treatment with a bronchodilator is often ineffective and the diagnosis of asthma in a young child should therefore be based on:

BOX 1.1   Diagnosing asthma

SIGNS AND SYMPTOMS OF THE CONDITION

Symptoms (episodic/variable)	Signs
• Wheeze	• None (common)
• Shortness of breath	• Wheeze – diffuse, bilateral, expiratory (± inspiratory)
• Chest tightness	• Tachypnoea
• Cough	

HELPFUL ADDITIONAL INFORMATION
- Is there a personal or family history of asthma or atopy (eczema, allergic rhinitis)?
- Is there a history of symptoms worsening after ingesting aspirin or other NSAID or after use of beta-blockers (including glaucoma drops)?
- Can the patient identify triggers – e.g. pollens, dust, animals, exercise, viral infections, chemicals, irritants?
- What is the pattern and severity of symptoms and exacerbations?

OBJECTIVE MEASUREMENTS
- Diurnal variation of > 20% in peak expiratory flow on 3 days or more in a week for 2 weeks, shown on a PEF diary
- Reversibility demonstrated by spirometry, the critical measurement being FEV_1 (forced expiratory volume in 1 second):
  - increase in $FEV_1 \geq 15\%$ (and 200 ml) after short-acting $beta_2$ agonist (e.g. salbutamol 400 µg by pressurised metered-dose inhaler (pMDI) + spacer or 2.5 mg by nebuliser)
  - increase in $FEV_1 \geq 15\%$ (and 200 ml) after trial of steroid tablets (prednisolone 30 mg/day for 14 days)
  - decrease in $FEV_1 \geq 15\%$ after 6 minutes of exercise (running)
- Histamine or methacholine challenge in difficult cases

BOX 1.2 Indications for referral for specialist opinion/further investigation*

- Diagnosis unclear or in doubt
- Unexpected clinical findings (e.g. crackles, cyanosis, heart failure)
- Spirometry results or PEF readings do not fit the clinical picture
- Suspected occupational asthma
- Persistent shortness of breath (not episodic, or without associated wheeze)
- Unilateral or fixed wheeze
- Stridor
- Persistent chest pain or atypical features
- Weight loss
- Persistent cough and/or sputum production
- Non-resolving pneumonia

*Consider chest x-ray in any patient presenting atypically or with additional symptoms.

BOX 1.3 Conditions to include in the differential diagnosis when asthma is suspected

- Chronic obstructive pulmonary disease (COPD)
- Cardiac disease
- Tumour:
  - laryngeal
  - tracheal
  - lung
- Bronchiectasis
- Foreign body
- Interstitial lung disease
- Pulmonary emboli
- Aspiration
- Vocal cord dysfunction
- Hyperventilation

- the presence of key features and careful consideration of alternative diagnoses
- assessment of the response to trials of treatment
- repeated reassessment of the child, questioning the diagnosis if management is ineffective
- a symptom diary, noting particularly nocturnal and exercise-induced symptoms and including a record of bronchodilator use.[1, 10, 11]

DATA CODING AND THE ASTHMA REGISTER

Once the diagnosis of asthma has been confirmed, in computerised practices the preferred Read code (H33) should be used to complete the patient's record.[1, 12] Patients who have chronic obstructive pulmonary disease (COPD) or no current evidence of asthma need to be coded appropriately or removed from the asthma register. An accurate register is an important tool to help ensure that asthma patients receive appropriate care and education. Guidance on creating a disease register

can be found in the *MIMS* GMS contract action plan.[13]

Under the new GMS contract, creating and maintaining an asthma register and diagnosing asthma using objective measurements can attract 22 quality points (Table 1.1). Other quality indicators for asthma are discussed in Chapters 2 and 3.

NURSE TRAINING AND SUPPORT

It is important that any nurse who diagnoses asthma has received adequate training and has support while working in an extended role. A survey of the role of the practice nurse in asthma

ACTIVITY

Can you produce an accurate register of patients in your practice with asthma?

Review the way in which your patients are diagnosed with asthma in light of the published evidence. Is there a regularly serviced spirometer in the practice? What new skills could you develop to implement change?

TABLE 1.1 Earning quality points for asthma care under the new contract

	Indication	Points	Payment stages
Records ASTHMA 1	The practice can produce a register of patients with asthma, excluding patients with asthma who have been prescribed no asthma-related drugs in the past 12 months	7	–
Initial management ASTHMA 2	The percentage of patients aged 8 years and over diagnosed as having asthma from 1 April 2003 where the diagnosis has been confirmed by spirometry or peak flow measurement	15	25–70%

management found that, although most nurses advise on inhaler technique with confidence, they are less sure about diagnosis.[14] As nurses we owe a legal duty of care to our patients, and are judged by the professional standard appropriate to the post we hold.[15] While working in an extended role, the practice nurse is therefore expected to operate at the skill level and with the competence expected of the GP or other professional who normally performs that role.

ACTIVITY

Consider your educational and legal accountability when undertaking an extended role in the management of asthma patients.

PREVENTION OF ASTHMA

While the exact cause of asthma is not clear, our present understanding of the disease suggests that it cannot be eradicated. It has long been known that a tendency to asthma and atopy runs in families, but the major role of environmental factors in the development of atopic disease is clearly indicated by the relatively low concordance seen among homozygotic twins. There is also a strong correlation between allergic sensitisation to common aeroallergens in early life and subsequent development of asthma.[16] However, more research will be needed before we can make effective interventions to reduce the incidence of asthma. Many environmental agents have been identified as possible risk factors, but different studies have yielded conflicting results and no precise relationship has been established between any proposed risk factor and the development of asthma.[10]

On the basis of current knowledge, however, there are several measures that practice nurses, our patients and society as a whole can implement, to promote the development of healthy lungs in children and reduce asthma exacerbations in those who have the condition.

Regular medication

Taking all prescribed asthma medication regularly, using the correct inhaler technique, is an important factor in preventing acute exacerbations. (The use of personal asthma action plans and annual reviews for people with asthma are discussed in Chapters 2 and 3.)

Upper respiratory tract infections

Respiratory infections are a common cause of asthma exacerbations. It is almost impossible to avoid catching them, but trying to steer clear of people who have a cold or flu and avoiding crowds may help. Advising patients not to touch their nose or eyes after they have been in physical contact with a person who has a cold, until they have washed their hands, may also be beneficial.

Influenza immunisation

Influenza is one of the few acute respiratory illnesses for which vaccination is available, and the Department of Health and the Joint Committee on Vaccination and Immunisation recommend that people with asthma should be immunised annually against influenza.[17]

Allergens and irritants

Avoidance of trigger factors, which include pollens, house dust mite, animal fur, fumes, certain foods, non-steroidal anti-inflammatory drugs (NSAIDs), stress and, most important, smoking, may help an individual with asthma to avoid exacerbations.

Tobacco smoke

Smoking is a recognised trigger of asthma, and the new GMS contract has focused heavily on reducing the number of patients who smoke. It is therefore important to ask about personal or passive smoking, advise smokers on the many adverse effects of smoking and offer support to those who wish to stop smoking. Smoking in pregnancy and maternal postnatal smoking have been proven to increase infant wheeze.[18]

Weather

Sudden changes in temperature and exposure to cold air and windy weather are common triggers for people with asthma. Taking an extra puff of a bronchodilator before going outside and wearing a scarf over the face in cold weather may help to minimise symptoms.

Weight reduction

Several studies have shown that obesity is associated with an increased likelihood of developing asthma.[19] Regular exercise and weight reduction are therefore recommended in obese patients to improve asthma control.

Breathing exercises

Buteyko exercises are a system of breathing exercises intended to reduce the rate and depth of breathing. Two studies have reported that some people with asthma who practised Buteyko exercises twice a day for 3 months needed less medication, but further research evidence is needed before we can recommend the exercises.[1] (See: http:// www.buteykohealth.com)

Breastfeeding

There is strong evidence that breastfeeding has a protective effect in relation to early-life wheezing.[20] It should be encouraged, and discussed with all pregnant women, particularly those with a history of atopy.

ACTIVITY

Suggest appropriate environmental public health strategies for the prevention of asthma.

CONCLUSION

Asthma is common in the UK and the condition is set to gain a higher profile as the new GMS contract is implemented. Nurses will be playing a key part in the detection and management of asthma in general practice, but should do so only after completing appropriate training and with the support of a GP or respiratory nurse specialist to whom patients can be referred when diagnosis is in doubt.

Practice nurses should be encouraged by the new BTS/SIGN guideline on the management of asthma, which provides comprehensive evidence-based advice for all health professionals with a role in asthma care.

EVALUATION ACTIVITY

Evaluate how successful any changes have been that you have made in your management of asthma patients on the basis of what you have learned in this chapter, from both a professional and a patient perspective.

LEARNING POINTS

- Asthma causes significant mortality and morbidity in the UK
- Susceptibility to asthma has a definite genetic component, but environmental factors also play an important part in development of the condition and exacerbation of symptoms
- The diagnosis of asthma is made on the basis of signs, symptoms, personal and family history, and objective measurement (PEF diary, reversibility testing)
- Long-term treatment with asthma drugs should only be started when other diagnoses have been excluded
- We do not yet know how to prevent the development of asthma, but measures can be taken that may reduce its likelihood and to reduce exacerbations in those who have the condition

---

REFERENCES

1. BTS, SIGN. British guideline on the management of asthma. Thorax 2003; 58 (Suppl 1): S1–S97. Available at: http://www.sign.ac.uk and http://www.brit.thoracic.org.uk
2. BMA and NHS Confederation. New GMS Contract 2003 – Investing in General Practice. London: BMA and NHS Confederation, 2003.
3. National Asthma Campaign. Asthma Audit 2001. Summary Factsheet 18 (updated September 2001). Available at: http://www.asthma.org.uk
4. McCormick A, Fleming D, Charlton J. Morbidity Statistics from General Practice. Fourth National Study 1991–1992. MB5 no. 3. London: HMSO, 1995. Available at: http://www.statistics.gov.uk
5. National Asthma Campaign. Asthma Audit 2001. Out in the open. A true picture of asthma in the United Kingdom today. Asthma J 2001; 6(3). Special supplement available from Asthma UK
6. GINA Report. Global Burden of Asthma, May 2004. Available at: http://www.ginasthma.com
7. Von Mutius E. Towards prevention. Lancet 1997; 350(Suppl II): 1417.
8. National Institute for Health and Clinical Excellence. Guidance on inhaler systems for under 5s with asthma. Technology Appraisal Guidance No. 10. August 2000. Available at: http://www.nice.org.uk/pdf/NiceINHALERguidance.pdf
9. International consensus report on the diagnosis and treatment of asthma. Bethesda, Maryland: National Heart, Lung, and Blood Institute, National Institutes of Health. Publication No. 92-3091, March 1992. Eur Respir J 1992; 5: 601–641.
10. PRODIGY Guidance. Asthma. Available at: http://www.prodigy.nhs.uk
11. National Heart, Lung, and Blood Institute. Guidelines for the Diagnosis and Management of Asthma. Expert Panel Report 2: 97–4051. Bethesda, Maryland: National Institutes of Health, 1997. Available at: http://www.nhlbi.nih.gov
12. National Health Applications & Infrastructure Services. Read Code Requests. Available at: http://www.nhsia.nhs.uk
13. MIMS GMS Contract Action Plan. Helping GPs Maximise their Clinical Indicator Payments. London: Haymarket Medical Publications, 2004.
14. Jones R, Freegard S, Reeves M, Hanney K, Dobbs F. The role of the practice nurse in the management of asthma. Primary Care Respir J 2001; 10(4): 109–111.
15. Bolam v Friern Hospital Management Committee 1957 (2 A11 ER 118, (1957) 1 WLR 582).
16. Lau S, Illi S, Sommerfield C, et al. Early exposure to house-dust mite and cat allergens and development of childhood asthma: a cohort study. Multicentre Allergy Study Group. Lancet 2000; 356: 1392–1397.

17. Department of Health. Immunisation Against Infectious Diseases. London: HMSO, 1996.

18. Cook D, Strachan D. Health effects of passive smoking – 10. Summary of effects of parental smoking on the respiratory health of children and implications for research. Thorax 1999; 54: 357–366.

19. Stenius-Aarniala B, Poussa T, Kvarnstrom J, et al. Immediate and long term effects of weight reduction in obese people with asthma: randomised control study. BMJ 2000; 320: 827–832.

20. Gdalevich M, Mimouni D, David M, et al. Breast feeding and the risk of bronchial asthma in childhood: a systematic review with meta-analysis of prospective studies. J Pediatr 2001; 139: 261–267.

Chapter 2

ASTHMA
Management of the new patient

Angie Heini

CHAPTER CONTENTS

LEARNING OBJECTIVES

After reading this chapter you will be able to:

- plan an education programme for a newly diagnosed asthma patient
- demonstrate the use of the common inhaler devices
- ensure that people with asthma who smoke receive appropriate smoking cessation advice
- use the preferred Read codes for data entry for smoking status

Some primary care teams may have tended to neglect their patients with asthma, because the lack of a National Service Framework targeted on respiratory disease has kept the focus on other chronic diseases. The publication of a new British guideline on the management of asthma and the quality points that practices can earn for asthma care under the new GMS contract are changing this. Practice nurses can play an important part in improving asthma management.[1]

SUPPORTING THE NEW ASTHMA PATIENT

The diagnosis of asthma can be frightening for a patient who has heard tales of people fighting for breath or even dying during an asthma attack.

The goal of the practice nurse should be to provide reassurance, by educating the patient about the condition and ensuring that his or her symptoms are relieved by appropriate medication. Structured care has been shown to produce benefits for patients with asthma, and as a practice nurse you should be introducing a standardised programme of care from the time of diagnosis.[2]

Education

Do not expect to complete the patient's education about asthma and its management at the initial consultation. Use of a wide range of approaches, such as discussion, demonstration, videos, leaflets and books, will help to ensure a successful patient education programme. Topics to be covered may include:

- information on the pathophysiology of asthma, to help the patient understand the condition
- information about trigger factors – avoiding common triggers such as tobacco smoke and animal dander can help prevent acute exacerbations (see Chapter 1)
- medication history – beta blockers (prescribed for hypertension, angina, arrhythmias and prophylaxis of migraine) are contraindicated in patients with asthma. Over-the-counter agents such as non-steroidal anti-inflammatory drugs (NSAIDs) may exacerbate symptoms
- the difference between 'preventer' inhalers that deliver anti-inflammatory corticosteroids and 'reliever' inhalers that deliver bronchodilators. Better patient understanding of asthma medication could save lives.[3] Poor understanding can lead to non-concordance with treatment, which is thought to contribute to 18–48% of asthma deaths[4]
- demonstration of inhaler technique – patients must use their device correctly for the prescribed drug to reach the airways
- common side-effects of asthma drugs – it is important that the patient knows what to expect in order to maximise compliance

- use of a peak flow meter – if regular measurements of peak expiratory flow (PEF) are needed to assess how well treatment is working, you will need to prescribe a meter and teach the patient how to use it
- the patient's health beliefs, and goals for the management of his or her asthma – it is important to establish an individual's attitude to asthma and the treatment needed
- how to recognise worsening symptoms and what to do in the event of a severe attack – written information is most effective
- negotiation of an asthma action (self-management) plan – such plans have been proven to significantly improve asthma outcomes.[5, 6] Examples of asthma action plans are available online from PRODIGY[7] and Asthma UK and are discussed further in Chapter 3[8]
- patients over 6 months old with asthma should receive an annual flu vaccination. This is recommended by the Department of Health and the Joint Committee on Vaccination and Immunisation.[9]

Remember that not all your information and leaflets need to be given at the first appointment – a progressive approach is much more likely to be effective. It is also important to take into account the patient's age, ethnic group, social status and any communication difficulties they may have, because education and advice are best tailored to meet the needs of each individual. Some patients may respond better to group education. Group sessions are organised by some asthma specialist nurses employed by the primary care trust (PCT) or could be offered in the surgery by practice nurses.

ACTIVITY

Investigate the availability of patient information leaflets about asthma in your practice and evaluate their content.

What further advice to patients do you think would be useful?

INITIATING TREATMENT

Nurses have an increasing responsibility in the management of patients with asthma and should be aware of the political and economic environment they are working in. This includes consideration of Government initiatives, such as the NHS Plan, the prescribing protocols of your PCT and your practice, and the availability of resources.[10]

Part of this extended role is consideration of the concerns of patients. For example, the British Thoracic Society/Scottish Intercollegiate Guidelines Network (BTS/SIGN) guideline recognises that the differing needs and expectations of asthma patients mean that fixed targets are not appropriate.[1] The practice nurse should help the person with asthma reach an informed choice about the management of their condition, based on a realistic assessment of the risks and benefits of treatment rather than on preconceived beliefs.

The aim of treatment should be to achieve early control of the patient's symptoms and so gain their confidence. Initial dosing therefore needs to be appropriate to the severity of the patient's asthma. Subsequently, the aim is to use the minimum amount of medication needed to maintain control. However, it can be difficult for inexperienced nurses to gauge the appropriate level of treatment, as there is no set starting dose or drug regimen. Nurses without appropriate training and skills should refer to a GP or respiratory specialist nurse for guidance.

The BTS/SIGN guideline suggests a stepwise approach to management, whereby patients at step 1 (adults and children of all ages with mild intermittent asthma) should use an inhaled short-acting beta$_2$-agonist as required to relieve symptoms.[1] Treatment steps 2–5 are discussed in Chapter 3. Always ensure that prescribing is in line with your practice protocol and your PCT's strategy for medicines management.

INHALER DEVICES

The key to efficient delivery of inhaled asthma drugs is the patient's ability to use correctly the chosen inhaler device. Compliance may be poor if the patient does not feel comfortable using a particular device. This means that their preferences should be considered, although this can be problematic if the medication required restricts the choice of device. The aim should be to gain control of the patient's symptoms with minimal medication (and minimal side-effects), with an easy to use device and a simple dosing regimen, at minimal cost.

With more than 90 individual inhaler products licensed for use in the UK, the choice of devices is almost overwhelming.[12] However, there are two main groups (aerosol and dry-powder – see Box 2.1), with different types suiting different people.

The choice of device for an individual depends on factors such as:

- convenience – will it fit into a pocket?
- coordination and manual dexterity – some devices need more than others
- personal preference
- devices available for the chosen drug
- age – children under 6 years old may not be able to use a dry-powder device effectively;

BOX 2.1   Inhaler devices available for the delivery of asthma drugs

Aerosol inhalers
- Pressurised metered-dose inhaler (pMDI)

Breath–actuated aerosol inhalers
- Easi-breathe
- Autohaler
- Syncroner

Dry–powder inhalers
- Accuhaler
- Diskhaler
- Spinhaler
- Turbohaler
- Twisthaler
- Clickhaler
- Cyclohaler
- Aerohaler

children under 12 years old and elderly people may not be able to use a pMDI without a spacer (see below).

The National Institute for Health and Clinical Excellence has produced guidance on the use of inhaler devices in children under the age of 5 years and in older children (aged 5–15 years).[13, 14]

ACTIVITY

Familiarise yourself with Section 3.1–3.3 of the *British National Formulary* (BNF).[11]

List the cautions for beta$_2$-agonists.

List the side-effects of beta$_2$-agonists.

List the drug interactions with beta$_2$-agonists.

SPACER DEVICES

Use of a spacer device with a metered-dose inhaler can improve drug delivery to the lungs and may be necessary for children, the elderly or those with poor inhalation technique. It is important to prescribe a spacer device that is compatible with the chosen inhaler (Table 2.1) and to consider the size of the spacer – larger ones may be more cumbersome but are the most effective.

It is vital that a competent healthcare professional assesses an asthma patient's ability to use an inhaler device. An alternative can then be found if the patient cannot satisfactorily use the device initially selected. An inhaler should be prescribed only when both patient and nurse are happy with the choice of device and the patient has received

---
ACTIVITY

Obtain as many different types of placebo inhalers and spacers as you can and practise demonstrating their use.

Consider how you would explain 'relievers' and 'preventers' to an asthma patient.

---

appropriate advice. A review appointment should be made for 1 month later to assess the response to treatment (e.g. if the patient is overusing their beta$_2$-agonist, treatment may need to be stepped up to control symptoms).

PATIENT ADVICE ON INHALER USE

- Do not exceed the prescribed dose.
- Follow the manufacturer's directions on inhaler use.
- If a dose of inhaled salbutamol (from the 'reliever' inhaler) fails to provide relief, obtain a doctor's advice as soon as possible.
- If you are changed on to a CFC-free aerosol inhaler, the dose may feel and taste different.
- Follow the cleaning instructions given in the patient information leaflet for each device.

SMOKING

It is important to ask newly diagnosed asthma patients about personal and passive smoking at the earliest opportunity and to offer support to smokers as appropriate. If there is not a nurse within the practice trained in smoking-cessation advice, then referral to a local specialist smoking-cessation clinic, if available, may be discussed with the patient. When patients decide that they want to stop smoking, use of nicotine-replacement therapy or buproprion should be encouraged, in conjunction with support. This has been

---
ACTIVITY

Is there a nurse in your practice with recognised smoking-cessation training?

Consider the training needs of all nurses within the practice.

Find out how to refer patients to your nearest smoking-cessation clinic.

TABLE 2.1   Spacer devices available for use with pressurised metered–dose inhalers (pMDIs)

Spacer	Type	Masks	Metered–dose inhalers
Able spacer	One piece, small volume (135 ml)	Infant, child, adult	Adapter allows fit to all MDIs
Aerochamber Plus	One piece, medium volume (145 ml)	Infant, child, adult	Adapter allows fit to all MDIs
Babyhaler	One piece, large volume	–	Compatible with Ventolin, Evohaler and Becotide
E–Z spacer	Collapsible, large volume (700 ml)	Silicone infant	Compatible with all MDIs; not prescribable at NHS expense
Fisonair	One piece, large volume	–	Compatible with Intel; not prescribable at NHS expense
Nebuchamber	Stainless steel, medium volume	Available from customer services	Compatible with Pulmicort; not available to prescribe or purchase on its own
Nebuhaler	Two piece, large volume (750 ml)	Paediatric	Compatible with Bricanyl and Pulmicort
Pocket chamber	One piece, small volume (110 ml)	Infant, small, medium, large	Adapter allows fit to all MDIs
Volumatic	Two piece, large volume (750 ml)	Paediatric	Compatible with Allen & Hanburys' MDIs

proven to improve long-term quit rates.[15] The new GMS contract has focused heavily on reducing the number of patients who smoke, allocating 18 quality points to the recording of smoking status (Table 2.2).[16]

In computerised practices the recommended Read codes should be used to record smoking status, so that the computer system can be searched to verify the practice's eligibility for payment (Box 2.2).

TABLE 2.2   Earning quality points for monitoring smoking status and encouraging cessation under the new GMS contract

Indicator	Points	Payment stages	Ongoing management
ASTHMA 3	6	25–70%	The percentage of patients with asthma between the ages of 14 and 19 years in whom there is a record of smoking status in the previous 15 months
ASTHMA 4	6	25–70%	The percentage of patients aged 20 years and over with asthma whose notes record smoking status in the past 15 months, except those who have never smoked, where smoking status should be recorded at least once
ASTHMA 5	6	25–70%	The percentage of patients with asthma who smoke, and whose notes contain a record that smoking-cessation advice or referral to a specialist service, if available, has been offered within the past 15 months

> **BOX 2.2   Smoking-related Read codes for use in computerised records**
>
> **Aerosol inhalers**
> - Never smoked: Read code 1371
> - Ex-smoker: Read code 137L
> - Smoker: Read code 137R
> - Smoking cessation advice: Read code 8CA

> **EVALUATION ACTIVITY**
>
> Think about the way in which newly diagnosed asthma patients are managed within your practice. What changes could you make on the basis of knowledge gained in this section?

CONCLUSION

Most people with asthma are treated in primary care, and practice nurses have a key role in guaranteeing that newly diagnosed patients receive appropriate care. The patient needs to have a full understanding of the condition, and to be able to recognise and act upon worsening symptoms. Nurses therefore need to develop their skills in patient education and regularly update their knowledge about asthma. They have a tough agenda if practices are to meet the targets set by the new GMS contract, but must also remember to ensure that asthma care remains patient centred.

> **LEARNING POINTS**
>
> - Education for the newly diagnosed asthma patient must be tailored to meet his or her individual needs
> - For asthma treatment to be effective, inhalers should be prescribed only after the patient's ability to use a device has been assessed
> - Smoking-cessation advice and support should be offered to all patients with asthma who smoke
> - If a practice is to gain maximum quality points under the new GMS contract, nurses need to use the recommended Read codes when recording patient information on computer

REFERENCES

1. British Thoracic Society, Scottish Intercollegiate Guidelines Network. British guideline on the management of asthma. Thorax 2003; 58(Suppl 1): S1–S97. Available at: http://www.sign.ac.uk and http://www.brit.thoracic.org.uk
2. Droogan J, Bannigan K. Organisation of asthma care: what difference does it make? Nursing Times 1997; 93: 45–46.
3. Carter S, Taylor D, Levenson R. A question of choice. Compliance in medicine taking: a preliminary review. Medicines Partnership, October 2003. Available at: http://www.medicines-partnership.org
4. National Asthma Campaign. Out in the open: National Asthma Campaign asthma audit. Asthma J 2001; 6(Suppl 3).
5. Gibson PG, et al. Self management education and regular practitioner review for adults with asthma. In: Cochrane Library 1999; issue 2. Oxford: Update Software, 1999.
6. Put C, van den Bergh PC, Lemaigre V, et al. Evaluation of an individualised asthma programme directed at behavioural change. Eur Respir J 2003; 21: 109–115.
7. PRODIGY. Guidance – Asthma. Available at: http://www.prodigy.nhs.uk/asthma
8. National Asthma Campaign. Be in Control Materials. Personal Asthma Plan. Available at: http://www.asthma.org.uk
9. http://www.doh.gov.uk/greenbook
10. Department of Health. The NHS Plan: A Plan for Investment. A Plan for Reform. Command Paper 4818-1. London: The Stationery Office, 2000. Available at: http://www.nhs.uk/nhsplan
11. BMA and RPS. British National Formulary 47. London: British Medical Association and Royal Pharmaceutical Society, March 2004; pp. 131–151. Available at: http://www.bnf.org
12. Haymarket Medical. MIMS for Nurses. London: Haymarket Medical, February 2004; pp. 148–163.
13. National Institute for Health and Clinical Excellence. Guidance on Inhaler Systems for under 5s with Asthma. Technology Appraisal Guidance No. 10. London: NICE, 2000. Available at: http://www.nice.org.uk/pdf/NiceINHALERguidance.pdf
14. National Institute for Health and Clinical Excellence.

Inhaler Devices for Routine Treatment of Chronic Asthma in Older Children (aged 5–15 years). Technology Appraisal Guidance No. 38. London: NICE, 2002. Available at: http://www.nice.org.uk/pdf/Niceinhalers_ldC38GUIDA.pdf

15. National Institute for Health and Clinical Excellence. Guidance on the Use of Nicotine Replacement Therapy (NRT) and Bupropion for Smoking Cessation. Technology Appraisal Guidance No. 39. London: NICE, 2002. Available at: http://www.nice.org.uk/pdf/NiceNRT39GUIDANCE.pdf

16. BMA and NHS Confederation. New GMS Contract 2003 – Investing in General Practice. London: BMA and NHS Confederation, 2003. Available at: http://www.nhsconfed.org/gms/default.asp

FURTHER INFORMATION

Asthma UK: useful source of information for patients: Tel. 020 7226 2260. Asthma Adviceline: Tel. 08457 01 02 03; http://www.asthma.org.uk

BMA and NHS Confederation. New GMS Contract 2003 – Investing in General Practice. London: BMA and NHS Confederation, 2003. Available at: http://www.nhsconfed.org/gms/default.asp

General Practice Airways Group (GPIAG): aims to promote best practice among all members of the primary care respiratory team. Membership is free for GPs; associate membership is free for nurses and other healthcare professionals. Tel. 0121 454 8219; http://www.gpiag.org

MIMS for Nurses: sent free, quarterly, to nurse prescribers; has useful practical information on the management of asthma: Tel. 020 8606 7500.

National Respiratory Training Centre (NRTC): accredited education and training for health professionals in conjunction with the Open University. Tel. 01926 493313; http://www.nrtc.org.uk

PRODIGY Guidance – Asthma. Available at: http://www.prodigy.nhs.uk/asthma

Respiratory Education Resource and Training Centres (RERTC): provides courses accredited by the University of Lancaster. Tel. 0151 529 2598; http://www.respiratoryert.com

Scottish Intercollegiate Guidelines Network: http://www.sign.ac.uk

Chapter 3

ASTHMA
Long–term management

Angie Heini

CHAPTER CONTENTS

LEARNING OBJECTIVES

After reading this chapter you will be able to:

- use the stepwise approach to the management of asthma
- negotiate an appropriate personalised asthma action plan with each patient
- audit the care given to patients with asthma in your practice

Asthma continues to have a major impact on patients' well-being and quality of life. The practice nurse has a fundamental role in increasing patients' expectations of their asthma control and delivering structured, yet individualised, care. Regular review has not always been common practice; often patients have been seen only during acute exacerbations of their asthma, with those overusing $beta_2$-agonists going unidentified. It is hoped that the British Thoracic Society/ Scottish Intercollegiate Guidelines Network (BTS/ SIGN) guideline on the management of asthma, together with the financial incentives offered to practices by the new GMS contract, will improve this situation.[1, 2]

INITIAL REVIEW

Following diagnosis and initial management (see Chapters 1 and 2), asthma patients should be reviewed 1 month after starting on a short-acting beta$_2$-agonist. In the case of people with asthma who are over the age of 45 years and smoke, it is worth reconsidering a diagnosis of chronic obstructive pulmonary disease (COPD), to ensure that they receive the most appropriate treatment. If there is any uncertainty about the diagnosis of asthma, or the patient has unexpected clinical findings, such as cyanosis, weight loss or chest pain, it is important for the nurse to refer the patient to a GP or asthma specialist nurse.

The initial review is an opportunity to continue the patient education programme (see Chapter 2) and to assess whether inhaled corticosteroids are necessary. In light of evidence from two recent studies that inhaled steroids can be beneficial in mild asthma, the 2004 update to the BTS/SIGN guideline recommends that inhaled steroids should be introduced in milder cases than previously recommended, i.e. considered for patients with asthma in whom any of the following apply:[3–5]

- exacerbation of asthma in the past 2 years
- using inhaled beta$_2$-agonists three times a week or more
- symptomatic three times a week or more
- waking one night a week.

The treatment of asthma varies from practice to practice and can be affected by factors such as a primary care trust's (PCT's) prescribing formulary. However, the evidence-based BTS/SIGN guideline recommends using a dose of inhaled steroid appropriate to the severity of the disease.[1] For many patients it is appropriate to start with beclomethasone 400 µg/day (200 µg/day for children), and step treatment up or down as necessary (Box 3.1).

Inhaled steroids

Patients may have concerns over the use of inhaled corticosteroids, and if concordance is to be increased it is vital that practice nurses address any misconceptions. When first prescribing a

---

BOX 3.1   Stepwise management of asthma in adults and children over 12 years of age (as recommended in the BTS/SIGN guideline[1])

STEP 1: mild intermittent asthma
- Inhaled short-acting beta$_2$-agonist as required

STEP 2: regular preventer therapy
- Add inhaled steroid* 200–800 µg/day, according to disease severity (400 µg/day is an appropriate starting dose for many patients)

STEP 3: add–on therapy
- Add inhaled long-acting beta$_2$-agonist (LABA)
- Assess control of asthma:
  - good response to LABA: continue LABA
  - benefit from LABA but control still inadequate: continue LABA and increase inhaled steroid* dose to 800 µg/day (if not already on this dose)
  - no response to LABA: stop LABA and increase inhaled steroid* dose to 800 µg/day
- If control still inadequate, institute trial of other therapies, e.g. leukotriene receptor antagonist or sustained-release (SR) theophylline

STEP 4: persistent poor control
- Consider trial of:
  - increasing inhaled steroid* dose up to 2,000 µg/day
  - adding a fourth drug, e.g. leukotriene receptor antagonist, SR theophylline, beta$_2$-agonist tablet

STEP 5: continuous or frequent use of oral steroids
- Use daily steroid tablet in lowest dose providing adequate control
- Maintain high-dose inhaled steroid* at 2,000 µg/day
- Consider other treatments to minimise the use of steroid tablets
- Refer patient for specialist care

*Beclomethasone dipropionate or equivalent.

'preventer' inhaler, give a detailed explanation of the risks and benefits of inhaled steroids and provide an information leaflet. It is also important to discuss, as appropriate, possible side-effects, such as:

- hoarseness, and candidiasis of the mouth or throat – this can be reduced if the patient uses a spacer (see Chapter 2) and rinses his or her mouth with water after using a steroid inhaler[6]
- adrenal suppression – patients on high doses should be given a 'steroid card'
- reduction in bone-marrow density following long-term inhalation of higher doses – ensure that the dose is no higher than necessary to keep the patient's asthma under good control
- growth retardation in children – the Committee on Safety of Medicines recommends monitoring the height of children receiving prolonged treatment with inhaled steroids.[7]

Asthma action plans

The Department of Health expects patients with long-term disorders to have the knowledge to self-manage everyday aspects of their condition, and to this end has set up the Expert Patient Programme, which is discussed further in Chapter 4.[8]

There is increasing evidence that those patients who have written, personal asthma action plans have improved health outcomes, and the benefit of using action plans in secondary care is well recognised.[9] The BTS/SIGN guideline recommends their use in general practice, although

there is less evidence of their effectiveness in primary care.[1]

You may decide to use a simple plan, developed in the practice, based on patients' symptoms or peak flow readings or both. Alternatively, you may choose a more elaborate pre-printed plan, including provision of an emergency course of steroid tablets; plans can be downloaded from the Asthma UK (formerly National Asthma Campaign) website or from PRODIGY.[10, 11]

In a recent study of patients' views of asthma and its treatment, 80% of respondents had never been provided with a written plan to guide them in making changes to prescribed treatment.[12] Importantly, once the use of a plan had been explained to them, 68% said they would find one helpful. This highlights the need for practice nurses to adopt a flexible, patient-centred approach to asthma management.

The aim should be to develop a management plan that is based on the patient's goals and lifestyle objectives, rather than solely on such goals as are typically set by health professionals, such as scores in objective lung-function tests. Patient involvement is fundamental to good asthma management and is discussed in Chapter 4.

PROFESSIONAL CONSIDERATIONS

Nurses taking more responsibility for the care of people with asthma must be confident and appropriately trained to review patients in an asthma clinic. They must receive adequate support for the extended role from the whole primary care team, and know their limitations and when and how to ask for help. If the nurse is to start or adjust treatment, the practice must develop a patient group direction (PGD) that conforms to Department of Health requirements.[13]

For many practice nurses the targets set by the clinical quality indicators of the new GMS contract will create an opportunity to take a lead, advance their roles and help their practice to maximise its income (Table 3.1).

ACTIVITY

Obtain and study various asthma action plans.

Devise your own management plan to suit your patients and practice.

Identify a patient with a recent acute exacerbation of asthma. In what ways might an action plan have helped prevent this attack?

Indicator	Points	Payment stages	Ongoing management
TABLE 3.1			Earning quality points for asthma management under the new GMS contract
ASTHMA 6	20	25–70%	The percentage of patients with asthma who have had an asthma review in the past 15 months
ASTHMA 7	6	25–70%	The percentage of patients aged 16 years and over with asthma who have had influenza immunisation in the preceding 1 September to 31 March

---

ACTIVITY

Reflect critically on the professional issues that a practice nurse needs to consider when caring for patients with asthma.

STRUCTURED REVIEW

The BTS/SIGN guideline highlights that a better clinical outcome is achieved for people with asthma if review of their condition is proactive and routine, rather than opportunistic or unscheduled.[1] However, primary care resources must be directed to patients with the greatest need. Instead of reviewing all asthma patients systematically, it may be necessary to concentrate on those who have had acute exacerbations, or who are using two or more beta$_2$-agonist inhalers a month.

An effective way to assess symptoms, and gain a subjective view of the patient's asthma, is to ask the three quality-of-life questions recommended by the Royal College of Physicians (Box 3.2).[14] As yet there are no Read codes to record the responses to these questions in the patient's record, but they complement objective measures used to monitor asthma, such as peak flow measurement, which can be misleading if taken in isolation.

To help identify those patients who would benefit from review, the three questions could be posed in a questionnaire attached to repeat prescriptions for inhalers. Other strategies that may help to increase concordance with asthma medication are discussed in Chapter 4.

STEPPING UP AND DOWN

Asthma patients need to understand that they have a variable disorder of the airways and that at times of exacerbation they may need additional treatment (see Box 3.1, steps 3–5). Before altering treatment, check compliance with existing therapies and reassess inhaler technique – never presume that a patient will continue to use an inhaler correctly.

Equally important as stepping up treatment when necessary is reducing inhaled medication to the lowest dose at which effective control of asthma is maintained. A survey found that almost 2.5% of patients could have their inhaled steroid dose stepped down after clinical review, and a recent randomised controlled trial indicated that this approach does not compromise symptom control.[15, 16] It is important to agree a review date with the patient to update the asthma action plan

---

BOX 3.2 Questions to assess an asthma patient's symptoms[14]

In the past month:

- Have you had difficulty sleeping because of your asthma symptoms (including cough)?
- Have you had your usual asthma symptoms during the day (cough, wheeze, chest tightness or breathlessness)?
- Has your asthma interfered with your usual activities, e.g. housework, work/school?

as necessary, to maintain effective management of his or her asthma.

When patients are identified who no longer experience symptoms, Read code 8793 (asthma step 0) can be used. An 'inactive' asthma register can then be developed, leaving those patients on treatment steps 1–5 on an 'active' asthma register.

ACTIVITY

How could you improve the uptake of annual asthma reviews in your practice?

PRACTICE PROTOCOL FOR ASTHMA MANAGEMENT

Nurses who undertake asthma reviews should use a protocol for the treatment and management of patients with asthma, so that the care is structured, effective and consistent. The protocol may also help protect nurses from claims of clinical negligence. Include the whole practice team when developing a protocol, because it is not only the practice nurse but also the receptionists, administrative staff, GPs and pharmacist who have an important role in ensuring seamless asthma care.

Organisational issues

The organisational aspects of a practice asthma protocol include:

- giving the name(s) of nurse(s) managing asthma care and a record of the completion of accredited diploma courses, such as those offered by the National Respiratory Training Centre or the Respiratory Education and Training Centres[17, 18]
- consideration of the necessary equipment, such as peak flow meters, spirometer, placebo inhalers and patient education materials

- list of Read codes that will be used in patients' records
- use of computer templates to guide diagnosis and management – are staff suitably trained?
- recall system – it is essential to have an active recall system, so that patients who do not attend can be followed up
- management of non-attenders
- where and when the patients will be seen – protected time and space for the nurse to run the clinic
- a review date for updating of the protocol in the light of new published evidence.

ACTIVITY

Discuss your role in the care of patients with asthma with the primary health care team.

What measures can you take to ensure that all members of the team are giving consistent advice?

IMPROVING ONGOING MANAGEMENT

There are various ways in which practices might choose to improve the ongoing management of their asthma patients. For example:

- conducting reviews by telephone or email. This is an effective method of increasing the uptake of asthma reviews, especially with busy patients and those who work full time.[19] Consideration of telephone consultations for routine review is now advocated by the updated BTS/SIGN guideline[5]
- effort by the primary care team to organise asthma care so that an equitable service is offered to all patients
- sharing of resources between a number of practices
- working with the pharmaceutical industry – e.g. using the expertise of their asthma specialist nurses for help with audit or running asthma clinics

- putting reminders on repeat prescriptions to make an appointment for asthma review
- running a monthly search for patients who are due for asthma review or using more than one beta$_2$-agonist inhaler per month
- identifying and contacting all patients with asthma who have not received their annual influenza vaccination; ensuring appropriate patients are up-to-date with pneumococcal immunisation[20]
- using appropriately trained healthcare assistants to check inhaler technique, measure peak flow and perform spirometry
- surveying patients to determine their views on their asthma care.

ACTIVITY

Implement two new ways of improving the care of patients with asthma in your practice.

Audit

For the first time primary care is being rewarded for the quality, and not solely for the quantity, of care delivered. For a practice to reap the benefits of the new GMS contract, both clinical care and the patient experience need to be recorded. Using a computer template when managing patients with asthma can standardise addition of data to the computer record, and make the delivery and audit of effective care much easier. The General Practice Airways Group has developed a set of respiratory Read codes that can be downloaded and used to fulfil the requirements of the new GMS contract.[21]

It is important to remember that simply running an asthma clinic does not guarantee high-quality care and that, as nurses, we need to evaluate the care we give to patients.

CONCLUSION

Effective management of asthma requires an ongoing partnership between patients and healthcare professionals. This can be achieved only with regular, structured review of all patients identified by an active recall system.

Practice nurses need a sound knowledge of the BTS/SIGN guideline on the management of asthma and the asthma quality indicators in the new GMS contract. This will help them to provide

---

ACTIVITY

Has an audit of asthma care been completed in the past year?

Using the computer, identify the number of short-acting bronchodilators and corticosteroids being prescribed in your practice, and compare this with the PCT average.

What percentage of your asthma patients have personal action plans?

EVALUATION ACTIVITY

Reflect critically on the current care of people with asthma in your practice, identifying strengths and weaknesses in the organisational system and in clinical care.

Update the practice protocol for the management of asthma patients in light of published evidence.

LEARNING POINTS

- The BTS/SIGN guideline provides comprehensive advice on asthma management
- Written asthma action plans should be discussed with each patient and a personal plan developed if appropriate
- Proactive, routine review of people with asthma results in better clinical outcomes than opportunistic management

high-quality care and record it in such a manner as to facilitate audit. They are in a position to bridge the gap between the patient perspective of good asthma control on the one hand and clinical guidelines and financially rewarded outcome measures on the other.

REFERENCES

1. British Thoracic Society, Scottish Intercollegiate Guidelines Network. British guideline on the management of asthma. Thorax 2003; 58 (Suppl 1): S1–S97.
2. BMA and NHS Confederation. New GMS Contract 2003 – Investing in General Practice. London: BMA and NHS Confederation, 2003. Available at: http://www.nhsconfed.org
3. O'Byrne PM, Barnes PJ, Rodriguez-Roisin R, et al. Low dose inhaled budesonide and formoterol in mild persistent asthma: the OPTIMA randomized trial. Am J Respir Crit Care Med 2001; 164 (8 Pt 1): 1392–1397.
4. Pauwels RA, Pedersen S, Busse WW, et al. Early intervention with budesonide in mild persistent asthma: a randomised, double-blind trial. Lancet 2003; 361: 1071–1076.
5. http://www.sign.ac.uk/guidelines
6. National Institute for Health and Clinical Excellence. Inhaler devices for routine treatment of chronic asthma in older children (aged 5–15 years). Technology Appraisal Guidance No. 38. London: NICE, 2002.
7. British National Formulary 47. London: British Medical Association and Royal Pharmaceutical Society, March 2004; p145. Available at: http://www.bnf.org
8. Department of Health. The Expert Patient: A New Approach to Chronic Disease Management for the 21st Century. London: DoH, 2001.
9. Hoskins G, et al. Do self management plans reduce morbidity in patients with asthma? Br J Gen Pract 1996; 46: 169–171.
10. http://www.asthma.org.uk/control
11. http://www.prodigy.nhs.uk
12. Haughney J, Barnes G, Partridge M, Cleland J. The Living and Breathing Study: a study of patients' views of asthma and its treatment. Prim Care Respir J 2004; 13: 28–35.
13. Department of Health. Patient Group Directions. Health service circular. HSC 2000/026. London: DoH, August 2000.
14. Royal College of Physicians of London. Clinical Effectiveness and Education Unit. Measuring Clinical Outcome in Asthma: A Patient-focused Approach. London: RCP, 1999.
15. Eveleigh M. The goal is for patients to be in control of their asthma. Nursing Pract 2002; 7: 21–23.
16. Hawkins G, McMahon AD, Twaddle S, et al. Stepping down inhaled corticosteroids in asthma: randomised controlled trial. BMJ 2003; 326: 1115.
17. National Respiratory Training Centre (NRTC): http://www.nrtc.org.uk
18. Respiratory Education and Training Centres (RETC): http://www.respiratoryetc.com
19. Pinnock H, Bawden R, Proctor S, et al. Accessibility, acceptability, and effectiveness of routine telephone reviews of asthma: pragmatic, randomised controlled trial. BMJ 2003; 326: 477–479.
20. http://www.doh.gov.uk
21. General Practice Airways Group (GPIAG): http://www.gpiag.org

FURTHER INFORMATION

Asthma UK: useful source of information for patients. http://www.asthma.org.uk

BMA and NHS Confederation. New GMS Contract 2003 – Investing in General Practice. London: BMA and NHS Confederation, 2003. Available at: http://www.nhsconfed.org

British Thoracic Society, Scottish Intercollegiate Guidelines Network. British guideline on the management of asthma. Thorax 2003; 58(Suppl 1): S1–S97. Available at: http://www.sign.ac.uk and http://www.brit-thoracic.org.uk

General Practice Airways Group (GPIAG): aims to promote best practice among all members of the primary care respiratory team. Membership is free for GPs; associate membership free for nurses and other healthcare professionals. GPIAG, Edgbaston House, 3 Duchess Place, Edgbaston, Birmingham B16 8NH; Tel: 0121 454 8219; http://www.gpiag.org

MIMS for Nurses: sent free, quarterly, to nurse prescribers; has useful practical information on the management of asthma. Enquiries to MIMS for Nurses, PO Box 270, Southall UB1 2WF; Tel. 020 8606 7500.

National Respiratory Training Centre (NRTC): provides accredited education and training for health professionals in conjunction with the Open University. NRTC, The Athenaeum, 10 Church Street, Warwick CV34 4AB; Tel. 01926 493313; http://www.nrtc.org.uk

PRODIGY Guidance – asthma: http://www.prodigy.nhs.uk

Respiratory Education and Training Centres (RETC): provides courses accredited by the University of Lancaster. RETC, University Clinical Department, Lower Lane,

Liverpool L9 7AL; Tel. 0151 529 2598; http://www.respiratoryetc.com

Scottish Intercollegiate Guidelines Network: http://www.sign.ac.uk

Chapter 4

ASTHMA
Promoting patient involvement

Angie Heini

LEARNING OBJECTIVES

After reading this chapter you will be able to:

- be aware of the expert patient programme and know about the local arrangements for patients with asthma
- understand how to tailor patient education programmes to individual need
- discuss ways of encouraging people with asthma to take responsibility for their own care
- provide a service that is accessible to all patients with asthma

Patients with asthma should not be passive recipients of treatment, but active consumers expecting good quality care in which they play a part. Many want a more constructive relationship with healthcare professionals, and a more personalised approach to their asthma management, but attitudes on both sides will need to change for partnerships to develop between health professionals and patients.[1]

Practice nurses have a crucial role in raising patients' expectations of quality of life, and helping them feel they are in control of their asthma rather than the reverse. They are ideally placed to encourage patients to take responsibility for managing their own condition and in this have the support of the Royal College of Nursing, which believes that partnerships with patients are key to the future NHS.[2]

EXPERT PATIENT PROGRAMME

Involving patients in healthcare has been Government policy for at least 30 years. Plans for an expert patient programme were announced in July 1999 and reaffirmed in the NHS Plan.[3, 4] *The Expert Patient* was published in September 2001. This is the report of a task force that included people living with long-term conditions, and representatives from the health and social care professions and voluntary organisations (such as the National Asthma Campaign).[5] A key recommendation was the introduction of self-management training programmes to help patients with a long-term condition develop the confidence and motivation to use information, professional services and their own skills to take control of their lives.[5] As a practice nurse you might consider using expert patient groups to help you manage more challenging patients and those who do not attend for regular review. The report states that expert patients:

- feel confident and in control of their lives
- aim to manage their condition and its treatment in partnership with healthcare professionals
- communicate effectively with professionals and are willing to share responsibility and treatment
- are realistic about the impact of their disease on themselves and their family
- use their skills and knowledge to lead full lives.

Asthma action plans

The Living and Breathing study concluded that implementing personal, written, asthma action plans is likely to raise low patient expectations about asthma treatment and help patients with asthma aspire to achieve their personal asthma goals[1] (for more information see Chapter 3). Enquiring about asthma patients' use of an action plan during any consultation will help lead to patients expecting to have one.

ACTIVITY

Contact the expert patient coordinator at your primary care trust (PCT) and find out if arrangements have been made for the delivery or commissioning of a user-led self-management programme for asthma.

In what way could you become involved?

The action plan approach is endorsed in the revised BTS/SIGN guideline on asthma management.[6] It does take a considerable amount of both the nurse's and the patient's time to develop a personal plan tailored to the patient's ability, lifestyle and attitude to asthma. You have to make each patient feel important, and help them not lose heart when difficulties such as literacy or language problems are a barrier to self-management. Consistency in patient care is enhanced if action plans are developed on a computer template available to any healthcare professional using the practice system.

PATIENT CHOICE

Patient preference is important in all aspects of asthma care – e.g. when selecting an inhaler device, or when changing treatment (see Chapters 2 and 3). However, there are other considerations. Effective medicines management should also minimise costs and make best use of health professionals' time.[7]

Nurses have increasing prescribing responsibility, and must consider the overall cost of care. They should also acknowledge that any change in management or treatment that a patient finds unhelpful is unlikely to be appreciated or adhered to in the long run. If it is your practice policy to write generic prescriptions for inhalers and a patient has a preference for a particular type, he or she could be encouraged to telephone different local pharmacies to find out where their favoured type is dispensed.

ACTIVITY

In what ways could the quality and outcomes requirement of the GMS contract be improved to fit in with patient choice and involvement? (Include the indicators discussed in Chapters 1–3.)

Increasing numbers of patients are using complementary and alternative treatments, such as acupuncture. There is insufficient evidence to recommend them, but if a patient believes that a treatment will help his or her asthma it is more likely to do so.[8] This might explain why herbal or homoeopathic remedies with no proven beneficial effects help some patient's symptoms.

Remember that patients have the right to choose whether to take medical advice, and some may opt for informed dissent. Appropriate recording of their choice, using Read code 9hA2, will ensure they are not included in the asthma targets for the new GMS contract.[9] Equally, non-attenders can be excepted if they refuse to attend for review. You may decide to use your recall system to send three letters, and then record non-responders using the exception Read code 9OJ2.

EDUCATION

The importance of education cannot be underestimated if we expect patients to participate in their own care (see Chapter 3). Establish whether patients can grasp complex medical information or need more basic facts. Either way, they need to acquire the skills and knowledge to take control of their asthma.

If patients are asked to measure their peak flow at home, for example, a nurse or healthcare assistant can help them develop skills in recording and interpreting readings. This should include demonstrating poor technique (e.g. not placing lips tightly around the mouthpiece) to show how this gives misleading readings. It is also worth pointing out that what counts as a 'normal' reading varies according to age, height and sex; otherwise concerns can arise if a meter is passed around the family.

Once use of a peak flow meter is understood, the patient should be alert to lower than usual readings as an early sign of loss of asthma control. How to recognise worsening asthma should be a priority for discussion.[10] Nurses have not always been good at explaining the early signs of a developing attack and when to seek urgent medical help. Always make sure – do not presume – that the patient has the necessary information.

Follow-up after an acute attack can help prevent a recurrence. Review treatment, and ask what the patient thinks was the reason for the attack. If the inhaler being used was empty, show how to check what doses are left; if inhaler technique is poor, consider a change of device.

REGULAR REVIEW

The target-orientated new GMS contract offers a financial incentive to perform regular asthma reviews (see Chapter 3).[9] In addition, these checks are an opportunity to develop long-term relationships with individual patients and build their understanding about their asthma.

Fixed targets are not appropriate in asthma management, because each patient has different needs and expectations to balance against the side-effects or inconvenience of treatment. Listen to the patient. Let them describe how their asthma has been since the previous consultation, and then ask specific questions to clarify issues such as compliance with medication. Does the patient think their treatment is helping? Discuss any problems with the prescribed inhaler device, as this is likely to be a key determinant of adherence.

Responses to questions about quality-of-life issues give a subjective view of the patient's progress. For example: 'How is your exercise tolerance, compared with last year?'

If you do not ask direct questions about activity levels the patient may not volunteer information, such as having to give up a physical job or no longer being able to play football with the children. Make it a priority to deal with areas of concern to the patient. A night-time cough, for example, may be troublesome to someone who has a demanding job and is not getting enough sleep, while cough with exercise may not be a concern if the patient has no interest in doing any.

It requires effort to explore each patient's attitude to asthma, but if patients learn to adjust their own medication or activities there is mutual benefit – future consultation time is saved and patients are free to get on with their lives. Beware of increasing health inequalities by spending extra time with assertive or demanding patients and those who bring lists of questions or volumes of website information, and neglecting needier or less articulate patients.

CONCORDANCE

Poor concordance with medication and review is common among people with asthma, and if you

---

ACTIVITY

In what ways could you involve patients in helping them to improve adherence to treatment?

What strategies may help improve patient compliance with medication?

---

appreciate the patient's concerns you are more likely to be able to help them.

Discuss any reasons a patient gives for failing to attend appointments. The patient may perceive no obvious or immediate benefit from treatment, or may not be motivated to take regular medication. Reasons for non-compliance include denial of asthma, treatment side-effects, severe stress or other priorities in life, alternative health views and drug or alcohol abuse. A study has suggested that poor knowledge of how asthma medication works, coupled with complex treatment regimens, can do more to reduce concordance than concerns about adverse effects.[11]

Sometimes compromise is necessary, such as changing to a once-daily dose of inhaled steroid, increasing the strength to allow fewer doses, prescribing combined therapy, or thinking creatively to come up with the best possible treatment. See Boxes 4.1 and 4.2 for some practical tips.

BOX 4.1   How to assess adherence to asthma treatment

- Prescription counting can give some indication of adherence to treatment
- Ask how often the patient forgets to take the medication
- Discuss patient attitudes to the disease and the practicalities of taking the prescribed therapy
- Assess level of symptoms and how often the reliever inhalers are used
- Ask the patient if they think their asthma treatment is helping

Source: National Respiratory Training Centre[12]

BOX 4.2   How to improve concordance with asthma medication

- Open-ended questions, like 'If we could make one thing better for your asthma, what would it be?' may help to elicit a more patient-centred agenda
- Make it clear you are listening and responding to the patient's concerns and goals
- Reinforce practical information and negotiated treatment plans with written instruction
- Consider reminder strategies
- Recall patients who miss appointments

Source: BTS/SIGN guideline[10]

ACCESS

The practice nurse needs to be accessible to patients with problems. This does not mean giving out your home or mobile telephone number, but you might need to consider new ways of contact. Possibilities include setting aside time for telephone consultations, as advocated in the updated BTS/SIGN guideline, or using fax or e-mail. Review by such means may be more popular with young adults, who are notoriously poor attenders, or people with difficulty getting time off work. Equally, elderly people and those in rural areas or who cannot afford public transport may appreciate not having to attend the surgery so often.[6]

If people are not attending your asthma clinic because they find the waiting room too noisy, or the clinic times inconvenient, or because they do not live on a bus route, such issues are likely to be a concern at other practices in the locality. Consider contacting the PCT to arrange clinics that fit in with patient needs, or a support group for people with asthma. You might also consider evening education sessions for asthma patients and their families, run separately to meet the needs of different groups, such as those from ethnic minorities or socially disadvantaged, elderly people or those with communication difficulties.

ACTIVITY

Arrange a survey of your patients to obtain their views on access to services for people with asthma.

How can you improve your service in light of the findings?

CONCLUSION

The practice nurse's key role in ensuring patient-centred asthma care is to educate people with asthma to recognise and act upon symptoms as recommended by the BTS/SIGN guideline on asthma management. Ideally this should be achieved through a partnership, in which the nurse has the knowledge to diagnose and treat asthma and the patient brings his or her personal experience of the disease and preferences with regard to its management. Both parties need to share information and make decisions jointly, recognising and respecting each other's area of expertise. Services for asthma patients must be accessible and fit around the needs and wishes of the patient, rather than those of service providers.

Practice nurses have the opportunity to empower a new generation of patients to take action to improve their health while looking to their healthcare professionals to be partners in their care.

EVALUATION ACTIVITY

Identify ways in which you can improve the involvement of patients with asthma in their care from the time of diagnosis.

Discuss your ideas with the primary healthcare team and set a date for implementation.

LEARNING POINTS

- Expert patients can change the delivery of asthma care and the relationship between clinicians and patients
- Patient education programmes must be tailor made for individual patients
- Patient choice is crucial in all aspects of asthma care
- Routine asthma reviews do not necessarily have to take place in the surgery

REFERENCES

1. Haughney J, Barnes G, Partridge M, Cleland J. The Living and Breathing Study: a study of patients' views of asthma and its treatment. Prim Care Respir J 2004; 13: 28–35.
2. Royal College of Nursing. Developing a National Plan for the New NHS: Nursing's Views on NHS Modernisation in England. London: RCN, 2000.
3. Department of Health. Saving Lives: Our Healthier Nation. London: Stationery Office, 1999.
4. Department of Health. The NHS Plan. Command Paper 4818-1. London: Stationery Office, 2000.
5. Department of Health. The Expert Patient: A New Approach to Chronic Disease Management for the 21st Century. London: DoH, 2001.
6. British Thoracic Society, Scottish Intercollegiate Guidelines Network. British guideline on the management of asthma: Update to printed guideline. Available at: http://www.sign.ac.uk/guidelines
7. National Prescribing Centre. A Guide to Achieving Benefits for Patients, Professionals and the NHS. Liverpool: NPC, 2002.
8. PRODIGY Guidance – Asthma. Available at: http://www.prodigy.nhs.uk
9. BMA and NHS Confederation. New GMS Contract 2003 – Investing in General Practice. London: BMA and NHS Confederation, 2003. Available at: http://www.nhsconfed.org/gms/default.asp
10. British Thoracic Society, Scottish Intercollegiate Guidelines Network. British guideline on the management of asthma. Thorax 2003; 58(Suppl 1): S1–S97. Available at: http://www.sign.ac.uk and http://www.brit-thoracic.org.uk
11. Carter S, Taylor D, Levenson R. A Question of Choice: Compliance in Medicine Taking: A Preliminary Review. Medicines Partnership, October 2003. Available at: http://www.medicines-partnership.org
12. National Respiratory Training Centre. Simply Asthma. A Practical Pocket Book, 6th edn. Warwick: NRTC, 2003.

FURTHER INFORMATION

Asthma UK (formerly the National Asthma Campaign): useful source of information for patients. http:// www.asthma.org.uk

Expert Patients Programme. http://www.ohn.gov.uk/ohn/people/expert.htm

MIMS for Nurses: sent free, quarterly, to nurse prescribers; has useful practical information on the management of asthma. Tel. 020 8606 7500.

PRODIGY Guidance – Asthma. http://www.prodigy.nhs.uk/guidance.asp?gt=asthma

Training providers

General Practice Airways Group (GPIAG): aims to promote best practice. Membership is free for GPs; associate membership is free for nurses and other healthcare professionals. Tel. 0121 454 8219; http://www.gpiag.org

National Respiratory Training Centre (NRTC): provides accredited education and training for health professionals in conjunction with the Open University. Tel. 01926 493313; http://www.nrtc.org.uk

Respiratory Education and Training Centres (RETC): provides courses accredited by the University of Lancaster. Tel. 0151 529 2598; http://www.respiratoryetc.com

DIABETES
Prevention and detection

Gwen Hall

LEARNING OBJECTIVES

After reading this chapter you will be able to:

- differentiate between type 1 and type 2 diabetes
- list the main complications of each type of diabetes
- describe the interventions that can be made to prevent type 2 diabetes
- plan a systematic approach to the prevention and detection of diabetes in primary care

The incidence of diabetes mellitus is increasing at an alarming rate – numbers are set to double within 25 years.[1] Currently around 3% of the UK population are diagnosed with diabetes, rising to 25% in Asian people aged over 60 years, and it is thought that a similar number are undiagnosed. Diabetes UK, the leading diabetes charity, promoted schemes to find the 'missing million'.[2]

There are two main types of diabetes: type 1 (previously referred to as insulin-dependent or juvenile-onset diabetes) and type 2 (previously referred to as non-insulin-dependent or maturity-onset diabetes).

- *Type 1 diabetes* occurs when the body either does not produce the hormone insulin or does not produce enough. Treated with insulin injections, required for life, type 1 diabetes tends to be managed through specialist or shared care.

- *Type 2 diabetes* occurs when insulin occurs when insulin production is reduced or when the insulin that is produced does not work properly (insulin resistance). Treated with diet and activity or tablets and/or insulin, the management of type 2 diabetes is shifting to primary care. Type 2 constitutes 85–95% of all cases of diabetes and it is this form that is largely responsible for the dramatic rise in the incidence of the disease.[1, 3]

There are some types of diabetes that do not fit easily into either of the two categories outlined above – e.g. type 2 diabetes of the young, gestational diabetes mellitus (GDM), slow-onset type 1 in the elderly. These conditions are explored in Chapter 7.

The aim of this chapter is to encourage you to plan a systematic approach to the prevention and detection of diabetes. We focus mainly on type 2 diabetes, as you are most likely to be involved in the care of patients with this condition.[4] We consider strategies relevant to primary care in line with the National Service Framework (NSF) for diabetes with a view to improving practice.[5, 6]

ACTIVITY
Why do you think the incidence of type 2 diabetes is increasing?

UPDATE ON DIABETES

There is no such thing as mild diabetes.

Type 1 imposes great strain on those who suffer from it and those who care for them. People with type 1 diabetes need daily insulin injections to survive and must control their blood glucose levels to maintain good health. When a person ingests carbohydrate, beta cells secrete insulin to help the body to use food for energy. If the pancreas does not make insulin or the body cannot use insulin properly, glucose builds up in the blood. Type 1 diabetes is thought to result from an autoimmune process causing the destruction of the insulin secreting beta cells in the islets of Langerhans in the pancreas.[7] This destruction leads to a rapid development of symptoms that require urgent treatment (Box 5.1).

With type 2 diabetes, the body either does not produce enough insulin (usually in slim people) or cannot use it properly (insulin resistance). In the latter case the beta cells work overtime to try to compensate for rising blood glucose caused by resistance to insulin. Blood glucose levels continue to rise and more insulin is secreted and so on until the beta cells become exhausted leading to secondary beta-cell failure (Figure 5.1). Once insulin resistance develops, glucose is forced into muscles and adipose tissues contributing to obesity and weight gain. Type 2 diabetes can take months or years to develop.

There are two schools of thought about what causes type 2 diabetes. One is that it is genetic. Studies of identical twins show almost 100% concordance – if one gets it, the other almost certainly will too. Even in the general population

BOX 5.1	Symptoms of diabetes
Type 1	Type 2
Rapid onset	Insidious onset
Often marked weight loss	May have weight loss
Hunger and/or abdominal pain	Pins and needles/ numbness in extremities
Type 1 and type 2	
Thirst	
Polyuria	
Vaginal thrush	
Changes to vision	
Lethargy/irritation	
Recurrent infections	

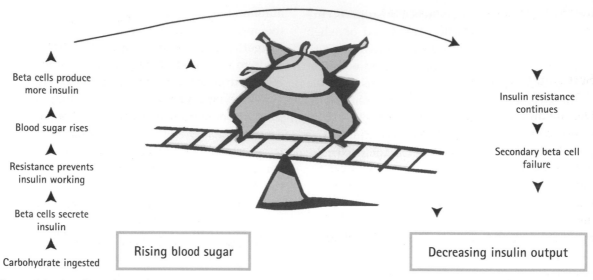

Beta cells produce
more insulin

Blood sugar rises

Resistance prevents
insulin working

Beta cells secrete
insulin

Carbohydrate ingested

Rising blood sugar

Insulin resistance
continues

Secondary beta cell
failure

Decreasing insulin output

Figure 5.1 Insulin resistance.

there is a positive family history in 30% of people with type 2 diabetes. The second school of thought is referred to as the 'thrifty gene' hypothesis – i.e. fetal malnutrition results in a decreased beta-cell mass, so insulin secretion in later life is inadequate to provide compensatory hyperinsulinaemia to combat the insulin resistance.[8]

Type 2 diabetes is known to affect older people, due to the progressive destruction of beta-cell activity associated with age, and certain ethnic minority groups (south Asian, African, African-Caribbean and Middle Eastern). The prevalence of type 2 diabetes is between three and six times higher in these populations compared with the white UK population.[5]

than 80 cm (32 inches) and men with waist measurements of more than 94 cm (37 inches) are at risk of developing type 2 diabetes.[9]

The first aim of the NSF for diabetes is to reduce the number of people who develop type 2 diabetes. Standard 1 of the framework states:

> *The NHS will develop, implement and monitor strategies to reduce the risk of developing type 2 diabetes in the population as a whole and to reduce the inequalities in the risk of developing type 2 diabetes.*[5]

The Government's 'five-a-day' programme promotes increased consumption of fruit and vegetables and increased levels of activity are being encouraged through the PE and Sport programme, community pilots for increasing physical activity,

PREVENTING DIABETES

At present, there is nothing that can be done to prevent type 1 diabetes. There are, however, a number of interventions that can be made to prevent the development of type 2 diabetes.[3] A lack of activity coupled with a high-fat diet producing a typical central obesity are known risk factors. Women with waist measurements of more

ACTIVITY
Find out what programmes and schemes exist locally to promote balanced diets, weight loss and physical activity.
Thinking about your area of practice, what could you do to encourage healthy living?

the Healthy Schools programme and local schemes such as exercise on referral.[6]

Screening for diabetes

Despite the increasing incidence of diabetes, there is no evidence to support screening the whole population. Having identified the causal factors of type 2 diabetes, however, it is clear that certain individuals may be more at risk than others and that early intervention might help to prevent the development of the condition (Box 5.2).[10] The most effective method of screening is yet to be established, but at minimum you need to adopt a systematic approach and work with all your colleagues in the primary care team.[5, 6]

DIAGNOSTIC CRITERIA

Diabetes is a man-made disease. That is to say we have fixed the criteria for diagnosis and, in response to research, the level at which it is diagnosed (Box 5.3). The level at which diabetes is confirmed has been lowered in response to research demonstrating that complications may be delayed or halted if detected early. The lower the diagnostic criteria, the earlier the detection.

Diagnosing type 1 diabetes is usually quite straightforward. The person is acutely unwell, perhaps ketotic, presenting with blood glucose results well in excess of diagnostic levels. The exception is slow-onset type 1 in the older, often slim, individual.

Any suspicion of diabetes in a child warrants urgent telephone referral direct to specialist care.

A person with type 2 diabetes may only be diagnosed after months or even years of increasing insulin resistance and slowly rising blood glucose levels. The 'deadly triad' of high cholesterol (typically hypertriglyceridaemia and decreased high-density lipoprotein (HDL)), hypertension and hyperglycaemia may already be present.[11] These factors, even without the

---

BOX 5.2   At-risk groups for screening

People with symptoms suggestive of diabetes
- Thirst, polyuria and weight loss
- Other urinary symptoms, such as nocturia, urinary incontinence
- Recurrent infections, particularly thrush (in women), skin conditions, foot problems
- Neuropathic symptoms, such as pain, numbness and paraesthesia
- Changes in visual acuity
- Vague or unexplained symptoms, lassitude
- Confusion in the elderly

People with conditions aligned to diabetes
- Hypertension
- Ischaemic heart disease
- Peripheral vascular disease
- Cerebrovascular disease
- Thyroid disease
- Polycystic ovary syndrome

People who are more prone to diabetes and who may warrant regular screening
- Those with obesity, particularly abdominal obesity
- People of Asian, African or African-Caribbean origin
- People aged over 65 years
- Those with a family history of diabetes or cardiovascular disease
- Women with a history of GDM or who have given birth to a large baby (birth weight > 4 kg)

---

raised blood glucose levels, have been shown to predict diabetes onset. Today, central obesity is added to that catalogue of risk.

Diagnosis must be based on a laboratory sample of blood, not on a reading from a blood glucose meter. No matter how well maintained, a meter will normally give a lower result, which may be falsely reassuring. If the person is asymptomatic but has a slightly elevated blood glucose result, you should repeat the test or perform an oral glucose tolerance test (OGTT).

BOX 5.3   Methods and criteria for diagnosing diabetes mellitus[11, 12]

- Diabetes symptoms (i.e. polyuria, polydipsia, unexplained weight loss) plus:
    - a random plasma glucose concentration ≥ 11.1 mmol/l *or*
    - a fasting plasma glucose concentration ≥ 7.0 mmol/l (whole blood ≥ 6.1 mmol/l) *or*
    - 2-hour plasma glucose concentration ≥ 11.1 mmol/l 2 hours after 75 g anhydrous glucose in an OGTT

- With no symptoms diagnosis should not be based on a single glucose determination. It requires a confirmatory plasma venous determination. At least one additional glucose test, on another day, with a value in the diabetic range is essential – either fasting, from a random sample or from the 2-hour post-glucose load. If the fasting or random values are not diagnostic, the 2-hour value should be used

---

The classifications impaired glucose tolerance (IGT) and impaired fasting glucose (IFG) are now seen as predictors of future risks:

- Impaired glucose tolerance (IGT) is a stage of impaired glucose regulation with a fasting glucose of < 7.0 mmol/l and an OGTT 2 hour value > 7.8 mmol/l but ≥ 11.1 mmol/l; it is a strong predictor for coronary artery disease.
- Impaired fasting glycaemia (IFG) is a level above the normal but below that diagnostic of diabetes, fasting venous plasma glucose > 6.1 mmol/l but < 7.0 mmol/l. This classification is considered a strong predictor for diabetes and Diabetes UK recommends that those with IFG should have an OGTT to exclude the diagnosis of diabetes.[12]

People diagnosed with either IGT or IFG should be offered advice about improving their diets and raising activity levels as part of a regular review process. The management of those newly diagnosed with diabetes is discussed in Chapter 6.

COMPLICATIONS

At the point of diagnosis approximately 65–70% of individuals with diabetes also have complications, such as coronary heart disease (CHD), hypertension and erectile dysfunction.[3] These complications are discussed in greater detail in Chapter 7, but some facts and figures are relevant here.

People with type 1 diabetes are susceptible to microvascular complications such as nephropathy, retinopathy and neuropathy. These conditions also affect people with type 2 diabetes, but for people with type 2 diabetes macrovascular disease is a more significant complication, with CHD accounting for over 70% of deaths – a complication that cannot solely be associated with age.[13] Overall, diabetes is still the principal cause of blindness in the working-age population and it accounts for most lower limb amputations.[15]

ACTIVITY

What percentage of your practice population are diagnosed with diabetes? If you have a large elderly population and/or a broad ethnic mix, you should have higher numbers. Does it meet the national average?[14]

Is there a call and recall system for those at risk of developing diabetes?

MANAGEMENT PLAN

Diabetes does not affect everyone in our society equally. There is a higher than average incidence of diabetes in lower socio-economic groups, who may have a poorer understanding of the risks and be less able to access appropriate services.[5, 6] In order to reduce the risk of developing type 2 diabetes in the population as a whole, as well as tackling the inequalities in the risk of developing this condition, the NSF for diabetes recommends the following key interventions:

- The overall prevalence of type 2 diabetes in the population can be reduced by preventing – and reducing the prevalence of – overweight, obesity and central obesity in the general population. This applies particularly to subgroups of the population at increased risk of developing diabetes, such as people from minority ethnic communities.
- Individuals at increased risk of developing type 2 diabetes can reduce their risk if they are supported to change their lifestyle by eating a balanced diet, losing weight and increasing their physical activity levels.

As a practice nurse, you are in an ideal position to coordinate efforts to implement a plan of action. Diabetes UK can provide posters and leaflets for the waiting room, highlighting symptoms and at-risk groups. Guidance has been issued on what constitutes a healthy eating plan (Figure 5.2).[15] Practice staff can be prompted, in many cases via computer systems, to check all those at risk of developing diabetes, and community nurses can assist with patients unable to attend the surgery. Call and recall systems can be put in place for those with a history of gestational diabetes, those identified as previously having IGT or IFG or those with a positive family history of diabetes. Community pharmacists are often keen to work in association with primary healthcare staff to promote healthy living.

CONCLUSION

Diabetes is rising to epidemic proportions, largely due to increasing numbers of people with type 2 diabetes. Even before diagnosis, risk factors and subsequent complications can be detected in around half of all cases.[4] Obesity, and in particular central obesity, is becoming a worldwide problem and as a healthcare professional you need to tackle this problem by actively promoting healthy living.

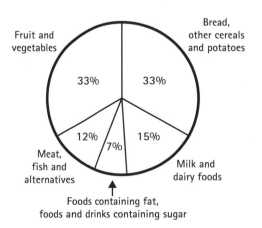

- Select a variety of foods from each group in the proportion shown
- Eat at least 5 portions of fruit and vegetables a day
- Eat foods containing fats and sugars sparingly and select lower fat options where possible
- Use less salt
- Drink plenty of fluid: 6 to 10 cups or glasses a day

Figure 5.2   Healthy eating plate.

> **LEARNING POINTS**
>
> - The incidence of diabetes mellitus is set to double within 25 years
> - Type 2 diabetes accounts for 85–95% of all cases of diabetes
> - Type 2 diabetes is largely preventable if individuals can be encouraged to eat a balanced diet, lose weight and increase levels of physical activity
> - More than 70% of people with type 2 diabetes will die of macrovascular complications, mainly CHD
> - A systematic approach to screening can help you to identify those at risk of diabetes and prevent or slow down the development of the condition

Diabetes is a costly disease, both to the patient and the NHS. We need to invest in preventive measures now to save in the long run.

EVALUATION ACTIVITY
Considering the evidence presented in this chapter, what changes could you make to your own practice to help prevent diabetes?
Consider links with other health professions in health promotion and dietetics.

REFERENCES

1. International Diabetes Federation. Facts & Figures. Available at: http://www.idf.org/home
2. Diabetes UK. Too Many Too Late. A Report. London: Diabetes UK, 2001. Available at: http://www.diabetes.org.uk/news/tmtl/report.htm
3. King's Fund. Counting the Cost of Type 2 Diabetes. London: Kings Fund/British Diabetic Association (now Diabetes UK), 1996.
4. Pierce M, Agarwal G, Ridout D. A survey of diabetes care in general practice in England and Wales. Br J Gen Pract 2000; 50: 542–545.
5. Department of Health. National Service Framework for Diabetes: Standards. London: DoH, 2001. Available at: http://www.dh.gov.uk/PolicyAndGuidance/HealthAndSocialCareTopics/Diabetes/fs/en
6. Department of Health. National Service Framework for Diabetes: Delivery Strategy. London: DoH, 2002. Available at: http://www.dh.gov.uk/PolicyAndGuidance/HealthAndSocialCareTopics/Diabetes/fs/en
7. Williams G, Pickup J (eds). Handbook of Diabetes. London: Blackwell Science, 1998.
8. Groop LC. Insulin resistance: the fundamental trigger of type 2 diabetes. Diabetes Obesity Metab 1999; 1: S1–S7.
9. Diabetes UK. Fact Sheet 22. Diabetes in Practice. Weight Matters. London: Diabetes UK, 2001.
10. Diabetes UK. Care Recommendation. New Diagnostic Criteria for Diabetes. London: Diabetes UK, 2000. Available at: http://www.diabetes.org.uk/infocentre/carerec/newdiagnotic.htm
11. Reaven GM. Role of insulin resistance in human disease. Diabetes 1988; 37: 1595–1607.
12. Diabetes UK. Recommendations for the Provision of Services in Primary Care for People with Diabetes. London: Diabetes UK, 2005. Available at: http://www.diabetes.org.uk/hcpreports/primary_recs.pdf
13. Joint British Societies 2005 Guidelines on prevention of cardiovascular disease in clinical practice. Heart 2005; 91: 1–52. Available at: http://www.diabetes.org.uk/hcpreports/heart.pdf
14. Audit Commission Report. Testing Times. A Review of Diabetes Services in England and Wales. London: Audit Commission, 2000. Available at: http://www.audit-commission.gov.uk
15. Department of Health nutrition forum. Available at: http://www.advisorybodies.doh.gov.uk/nutritionforum/index.htm

FURTHER INFORMATION

British Heart Foundation: has a wealth of free literature and leaflets for the public and health professionals that can be ordered easily online. http://www.bhf.org.uk

British Hypertension Society has a list of accredited electronic blood pressure devices and up to date information for patients and professionals: http://www.bhsoc.org

Diabetes UK: the leading charity for diabetes in the UK. The Diabetes UK website has areas for people with diabetes and health professionals. http://www.diabetes.org.uk

National Institute for Health and Clinical Excellence: has published management guidelines for type 2 diabetes on blood pressure, lipids, glucose, renal and retinopathy. http://www.nice.org.uk

National Service Framework for Diabetes: builds on and links with other NSFs, such as that for CHD and Older People. Department of Health, NSF website: http://www.dh.gov.uk/PolicyAndGuidance/HealthAndSocialCareTopics/Diabetes/fs/en

Chapter 6

DIABETES
Management of the new patient

Gwen Hall

LEARNING OBJECTIVES

After reading this chapter you will be able to:

- discuss the advantages of a systematic approach to the care of people newly diagnosed with diabetes
- provide up-to-date advice on nutrition
- list targets for metabolic control and the control of cardiovascular risk factors in people with diabetes
- describe common medical emergencies that may affect a person presenting with diabetes

The key to success in the management of diabetes is a systematic approach. As soon as diagnosis is confirmed (see Chapter 5) the person concerned should be placed on a practice diabetes register and encouraged to participate in a flexible education programme, which can be tailored to meet individual needs, to help the person and his

ACTIVITY

How do you help new patients with diabetes to understand and manage the condition?

List three areas you do well in and three you would like to improve.

or her carers take control of the management of the condition.

The National Service Framework (NSF) for Diabetes Delivery Strategy suggests that people with diabetes should have a personal diabetes record that:[1]

- includes an agreed care plan, including education and the personal goals of the person with diabetes
- sets out how their diabetes is to be managed until their next review to foster greater understanding and ownership of the goals of diabetes care
- identifies health, social care and education needs, how they will be met and who will be responsible
- identifies the named contact.

One of the two critical diabetes-specific targets, set out in the planning and performance framework for the NHS for 2003–2006, is for primary care to update practice-based registers so that:

Patients with CHD and diabetes continue to receive appropriate advice and treatment in line with NSF standards and, by March 2006, ensure practice-based registers and systematic treatment regimes, including appropriate advice on diet, physical activity and smoking, also cover the majority of patients at high risk of CHD, particularly those with hypertension, diabetes and a body mass index (BMI) greater than 30.[2]

Drawing on the NSF for diabetes, the aim of this chapter is to outline a systematic approach to the management of people who have been newly diagnosed with diabetes and who are being supported by primary care. Early interventions to prevent complications through control of blood glucose, blood pressure and lipids will also be considered.

For people with type 2 diabetes it is important to consider lifestyle interventions – healthy eating, weight loss, increased activity and smoking cessation – before resorting to medication.

DIET OR NUTRITION? EXERCISE OR ACTIVITY?

For many people the word 'diet' has unfortunate associations with failed attempts at slimming. For this reason, the terms 'nutrition' and 'healthy eating' are to be preferred. As a nation we consume less calories than 20 years ago, but we weigh more because we are less active.[3]

All people with newly diagnosed diabetes should have access to appropriate advice on healthy eating – preferably from a dietitian. As a practice nurse, however, you are likely to be the first point of contact for the patient and so must keep up to date with rapidly changing dietary information and advice. The Nutrition Subcommittee of the Diabetes Care Advisory Committee of Diabetes UK has updated its advice on nutrition.[4] Important changes include:

- greater flexibility in the amount of carbohydrate and monounsaturated fat as part of a balanced diet
- further liberalisation in the consumption of sucrose – provided it is eaten in the context of a healthy diet and distributed throughout the day
- more active promotion of foods with a low glycaemic index
- greater emphasis on the provision of nutritional advice in the context of wider lifestyle changes, particularly physical activity.

The glycaemic index is intended to identify foods that have a less marked effect on blood glucose levels (low glycaemic index) and those that cause a rise (high glycaemic index). You are advised to acquaint yourself with the detail of the recommendations to ensure that you are providing the best possible nutritional advice and information. The current recommendations on dietary composition are summarised in Table 6.1.

Nutritional advice and information cannot be delivered as a standard package together with education about other lifestyle issues. Rather it should be provided as part of an ongoing, interactive process that is responsive to individual needs. This will be reflected in the agreed care plan and goals set in the personal diabetes record.

THE VALUE OF CONTROL

Two large-scale studies have demonstrated the value of control in diabetes. The Diabetes Control and Complications Trial (DCCT) showed that retinal and renal complications could be halted or even prevented in type 1 diabetes if tight blood glucose control was maintained.[5] The United Kingdom Prospective Diabetes Study (UKPDS) found that tight control of blood glucose levels also helped to reduce the risk of microvascular disease in patients with type 2 diabetes and, most significantly, that tight control of blood pressure reduced the risk of any non-fatal and fatal diabetic complications and of death related to diabetes.[6]

ACTIVITY

How far does the nutritional advice and information you provide for people with diabetes reflect the recommendations made by the Nutrition Subcommittee?

Do you provide people newly diagnosed with diabetes with written information summarising the key dietary messages that they can take home and refer to later?

TABLE 6.1   The composition of the diet[4]

Component	Comment
Protein	Not > 1 g per kg body weight
Total fat	< 35% of energy intake
Saturated and transunsaturated fat	< 10% of energy intake
n-6 polyunsaturated fat	< 10% of energy intake
n-3 polyunsaturated fat	Eat fish, especially oily fish, once or twice weekly. Fish-oil supplements are not recommended
cis-Monounsaturated fat	10–20% } 60–70% of energy intake
Total carbohydrate	45–60%
Sucrose	Up to 10% of daily energy, provided it is eaten in the context of a healthy diet. Those who are overweight or who have hypertriglyceridaemia should consider using non-nutritive sweeteners where appropriate
Fibre	No quantitative recommendation
	Soluble fibre – has beneficial effects on glycaemic and lipid metabolism
	'Insoluble' fibre – no direct effects on glycaemic and lipid metabolism but its high satiety content may benefit those trying to lose weight and it is advantageous to gastrointestinal health
Vitamins and antioxidants	Encourage foods naturally rich in vitamins and antioxidants. With the exception of some patients in 'special groups' and 'special situations' there is no evidence for the use of supplements and some evidence that some are harmful
Salt	≥ 6 g sodium chloride per day

Blood glucose control

DCCT and UKPDS were landmarks in diabetes control and have resulted in tight targets for day-to-day blood glucose control and longer term management through laboratory tests (HbA_{1c}). As the majority of your diabetes patients will have type 2 diabetes, we focus here on guidance issued by the National Institute for Health and Clinical Excellence (NICE)[3] for the management of this condition, but do remember that the microvascular complications of type 1 diabetes also require diligent metabolic control (Table 6.2).[7]

An HbA_{1c} (glycosylated haemoglobin) test measures a person's average blood glucose (sugar) level for the 2–3 month period before the test. It can be used to assess the patient's condition and the need for change of treatment, and should form part of the care plan. Type 2 diabetes is a progressive condition and results will rise with time. Continual assessment and review will help to ensure that potential problems are highlighted, and treated, at an early stage.

Self-monitoring

There is great debate as to whether people with diabetes should monitor their own blood glucose levels.[8] The Audit Commission found that

TABLE 6.2 Recommendations for the provision of services in primary care for people with diabetes[7]		
	Desirable targets for people with type 1 diabetes	Desirable targets for people with type 2 diabetes
HDA_{1c} (DCCT standardised)	≤ 6.5% (but ≤ 7.5% for those at risk of sever hypoglycaemia)	
Self-monitored blood glucose (mmol/l)		
Fasting/preprandial	5.1–6.5 (whole blood) 5.7–7.3 (plasma)	< 5.5 (whole blood) < 6.2 (plasma)
Postprandial (2 hours after food)	7.6–9.0 (whole blood) 8.5–10.1 (plasma)	< 7.5 (whole blood) < 8.4 (plasma)
Before going to bed	6.0–7.5 (whole blood) 6.7–8.4 (plasma)	– –
Blood pressure (mmHg)		
Normal albumin excretion rate	< 135/85	< 140/80
Abnormal albumin excretion rate	< 130/80	< 135/75
Lipids		
Total cholesterol	< 5 mmol/l	
LDL cholesterol	< 2.6 mmol/l	
HDL cholesterol	≥ 1.0 mmol/l for men ≥ 1.2 mmol/l for women	
Triglycerides	≤ 2.3 mmol/l	
Body mass index (kg/m²)	< 25.0 for caucasians < 23.0 for those from an Asian background	

patients may not be clear about why they are encouraged to do so:[9]

> I have no idea whatsoever why I do daily blood-checks ... I have not the remotest idea what I am keeping the record for.

NICE concludes that for people with type 2 diabetes, self-monitoring:

- should not be considered as a stand-alone intervention
- should be taught if the need/purpose is clear and agreed with the patient
- can be used in conjunction with appropriate therapy as part of integrated self-care.[2]

People with type 1 diabetes, however, may need to test blood glucose levels several times each day to adjust their insulin levels and prevent hypoglycaemia (see Chapter 7). The NSF for diabetes emphasises the importance of involving patients in decisions about their diabetes.[1] For self-monitoring to be useful, both you and your patient need to be clear about what you hope to achieve by testing blood glucose levels.

For most people, most of the time, blood glucose levels should be maintained at around 4–8 mmol/l and HbA_{1c} levels at 6.5–7%, but 'normal' levels depend on individual circumstances.

For a person with type 2 diabetes who is asymptomatic and prepared to make lifestyle changes, your aim will be to help reduce blood glucose levels to as near normal as possible. You, your patient, and your primary care colleagues, may decide to try lifestyle interventions for 3 months before considering pharmacological interventions. For a person with symptoms, significantly elevated blood glucose and HbA_{1c} levels and with little capacity for making lifestyle changes you may consider medication at the outset.

Beware the slim patient newly diagnosed with type 2 diabetes – a history of weight loss may indicate poor beta-cell function and insulin therapy may be required. An HbA_{1c} test after 3 months will tell you how the patient is doing. Oral hypoglycaemic agents and insulin are considered in Chapter 7.

Blood pressure

Blood glucose control should not be considered in isolation. Many people newly diagnosed with diabetes will already be hypertensive. As UKPDS demonstrated, good blood pressure control significantly reduces the risk of CHD – the highest cause of mortality in type 2 diabetes. Any overall reduction in blood pressure reduces the risk of complications and will, therefore, have a huge impact on future quality of life.

NICE emphasises the importance of assessing and managing cardiovascular risk (Box 6.1) and this applies to all your patients but especially those newly diagnosed with type 2 diabetes.[11] These patients may have an opportunity to help themselves by eating a healthy diet, losing weight, increasing physical activity and giving up smoking. Pharmacological interventions should only be considered if, despite lifestyle changes, the blood pressure remains elevated on three occasions over 2 months.

The Joint British Societies Guidelines[12] recommend treating all people with type 2 diabetes as 'coronary equivalents' and no longer advocate calculating their 10-year risk. The advice is to manage all metabolic abnormalities with a holistic approach.

BOX 6.1   10-year coronary event risk[11]

A person at higher risk is one:
- who has manifest cardiovascular disease (a history or symptoms of coronary heart disease, stroke or peripheral vascular disease) *or*
- whose 10-year coronary event risk is assessed as above 15%, taking into account the known limitations of risk assessment charts

A person at lower risk is one:
- who does not have manifest cardiovascular disease
- whose 10-year coronary event risk is 15% or below, taking into account the known limitations of risk assessment charts

---

Lipids

High blood lipid levels contribute to CHD risk. This risk can be reduced by lipid-lowering medication combined with healthy eating and an active lifestyle. At diagnosis, fasting lipids should be checked and, if raised, re-evaluated after 3 months (see Table 6.2). Other factors that may abnormally affect lipids should be checked:

- alcohol consumption
- thyroid function to exclude hypothyroidism
- liver function to exclude liver disease
- creatinine and microalbumin to exclude kidney disease.

Pharmacological intervention is outlined in the NICE guidance which should be consulted before offering drug therapy.[11]

ACTIVITY

Do you have an agreed care plan for blood glucose, blood pressure and lipids for people with diabetes?

What targets do you use for those of ethnic origin?

How do you involve people with diabetes in the decision-making process to encourage them to take their medication?

COMMON MEDICAL EMERGENCIES

As the type of medical emergencies that occur in those newly diagnosed, or undiagnosed, with diabetes usually warrant urgent admission to hospital, you are unlikely to encounter them in day-to-day practice. You should however be aware of the presenting features.

Diabetic ketoacidosis

This is still the highest cause of death in young people with type 1 diabetes. They can present with diabetic ketoacidosis, having been increasingly unwell over a short period. Symptoms develop rapidly and within a day or two the person is acutely ill. Blood glucose levels are usually over 25 mmol/l, but may be lower. As the body attempts to rid itself of excess glucose by passing it out in the urine, dehydration is marked. Toxicity leads to general malaise, nausea and vomiting, sometimes accompanied by abdominal pain. If allowed to continue, confusion will set in with gradual loss of consciousness and, ultimately, coma. Some people can detect acetone on the breath, said to smell like pear drops. Diagnosis can be confirmed by detection of glucose and ketones in the urine. Diabetic ketoacidosis requires urgent treatment.

Hyperosmolar non-ketotic coma (HONK)

This condition presents in older people with type 2 diabetes, either previously undiagnosed or untreated, and is the result of prolonged hyperglycaemia. Again, dehydration is marked but there may be only low levels of ketones in the urine or none at all. Symptoms – thirst, oliguria, irritability – develop over days or even weeks, culminating in confusion, seizures or coma. The risk of coma is increased in patients taking drugs such as phenytoin, propranolol, cimetidine, thiazide or loop diuretics, corticosteroids or chlorpromazine.[12]

CONCLUSION

With type 1 diabetes insulin therapy is required immediately and for life. With type 2 diabetes there is an opportunity for patients to make lifestyle changes that may halt or slow down the progression of the disease if interventions can be made at an early stage. By instigating a planned and systematic approach to diabetes management you can help your patients to improve the quality of their lives both now and in the future.

EVALUATION ACTIVITY	LEARNING POINTS
How do you help people newly diagnosed with diabetes to decide whether to monitor their own blood glucose levels? What do you do with the results? Can you think of reasons why self-monitoring may not be effective?	• It is important to find approaches to the management of diabetes that are likely to be adhered to and that give the best chance of success • Systematic blood glucose, lipid and blood pressure control lessens complications • Patient involvement is key to good metabolic control • With type 2 diabetes lifestyle interventions made at an early stage may halt or slow down the progression of the disease

REFERENCES

1. Department of Health. National Service Framework for Diabetes: Standards and Delivery Strategy. London: DoH, 2002. Available at: http://www.dh.gov.uk/PolicyAndGuidance/HealthAndSocialCareTopics/Diabetes/fs/en
2. Department of Health. Improvement, Expansion and Reform. The Next Three Years' Priorities and Planning Framework, 2003–2006. Appendix B . Available at: http://www.dh.gov.uk/PublicationsAndStatistics/Publications/PublicationsPolicyAndGuidance/PublicationsPolicyAndGuidanceArticle/fs/en?CONTENT_ID=4008430&chk=lXp8vH
3. National Institute for Health and Clinical Excellence. Management of Type 2 Diabetes. Management of Blood Glucose. Inherited Guideline G. London: NICE, 2002. Available at: http://www.nice.org.uk/page.aspx?o=GuidelineG
4. Nutrition Subcommittee of the Diabetes Care Advisory Committee of Diabetes UK. The implementation of nutritional advice for people with diabetes. Diabet Med 2003; 20: 786–807. Available at: http://www.diabetes.org.uk/infocentre/carerec/nutrition.pdf
5. Diabetes Control and Complications Trial (DCCT) Research Group. The effect of intensive treatment of diabetes on the development and progression of long-term complications in insulin-dependent diabetes mellitus. N Engl J Med 1993; 329: 977–986.
6. United Kingdom Prospective Diabetes Study. Tight blood pressure control and risk of macrovascular and microvascular complications in type 2 diabetes: (UKPDS 38). BMJ 1998; 317: 703–713.
7. Diabetes UK. Recommendations for the Provision of Services in Primary Care for People with Diabetes.London: Diabetes UK, 2005. Available at: http://www.diabetes.org.uk/hcpreports/primary_recs.pdf
8. National Prescribing Centre. When and how should patients with diabetes mellitus test blood glucose? MeReC Bull 2002; 13(1): 1–4. Available at: http://www.npc.co.uk/MeReC_Bulletins/2002Volumes/vol13no1.pdf
9. Audit Commission. Testing Times. A Review of Diabetes Services in England and Wales. London: Audit Commission, 2002. Available at: http://www.audit-commission.gov.uk/Products/NATIONAL-REPORT/EB2CA6BA-C5E5-4B8F-A984-898D19E8C603/nrdiabet.pdf
10. Owens D, Barnett AH, Pickup J, et al. The continuing debate on self-monitoring of blood glucose. Diabetes Primary Care 2005; 6(1): 9–21.
11. National Institute for Health and Clinical Excellence. Management of Type 2 Diabetes. Management of Blood Pressure and Blood Lipids. Inherited Guideline H. London: NICE, 2002. Available at: http://www.nice.org.uk/page.aspx?o=GuidelineH
12. Joint British Societies. Guidelines on prevention of cardiovascular disease in clinical practice. Heart 2005; 91: 1–52.
13. National Patients' Access Team. GP Emergency Guidelines. September 2001.

FURTHER INFORMATION

British Heart Foundation: has practical leaflets, especially the Health Information Series, on lipid control and many other aspects of CHD. These are available to the public and health professionals online at: http://www.bhf.org.uk

Diabetes UK: has a wealth of leaflets, both free and for sale, to assist with your management of newly diagnosed patients. You can join as a professional member to receive journals and magazines to keep informed of diabetes care and research developments and advance notice of conferences. Diabetes UK, 10 Parkway, London NW1 7AA. Tel. 020 7424 1000; http://www.diabetes.org.uk

MacKinnon M. Providing Diabetes Care in General Practice, 4th edn. London: Class Publishing, 2002. A practical guide to diabetes in primary care. Plans for initial and ongoing management are clearly discussed.

National Institute for Health and Clinical Excellence (NICE): has issued guidance on blood glucose control, blood pressure and lipid control, screening for renal disease and retinopathy. Available at: http://www.nice.org.uk

National Service Framework: examples of good practice in changing services are identified on the NSF for diabetes website at: http://www.dh.gov.uk/PolicyAndGuidance/ HealthAndSocialCareTopics/Diabetes/fs/en

DIABETES
Long–term management

Gwen Hall

LEARNING OBJECTIVES

After reading this chapter you will be able to:

- plan systematic review for all patients on your diabetes register
- describe current guidance on blood glucose control
- list the main classes of oral hypoglycaemic agents
- outline the mode of action of commonly used insulins
- access sources of information and national guidelines via the worldwide web

In Chapters 5 and 6 we discussed the prevention, detection and early management of diabetes mellitus. We have learnt that type 1 disease (previously known as insulin-dependent or juvenile-onset diabetes) accounts for around 15% of all cases, with most of these managed through specialist or shared care. Type 2 disease (previously known as non-insulin-dependent or maturity-onset diabetes) presents a challenge to primary care.

Type 2 diabetes is a very serious condition. It has a huge impact on individuals who live with it and on their relatives and carers. Life expectancy is reduced; mortality rates from coronary heart disease may be five times higher and risk of stroke three times higher. It is a leading cause of kidney failure and of blindness, and accounts for many lower-limb amputations.[1]

Prevention, early detection, education and systematic management are the keys to success with diabetes. In this chapter we consider long-term management of diabetes and pharmaceutical intervention. Current advice on oral agents and insulin is included, with links to key documents highlighted for further study. Some less common forms of diabetes are outlined.

ACTIVITY

Why do you think type 2 diabetes is predominantly managed within primary care when type 1 in its early stages has fewer complications?

PLANNING A SYSTEMATIC APPROACH

Large studies have shown that good metabolic control is crucial to the prevention of complications in diabetes. Systematic review makes good control an achievable target for all people with diabetes and must include:[2, 3]

- An effective diabetes register. This is a critical element of the National Service Framework (NSF) for diabetes.[1] A target of March 2006 was set for these registers to be used to facilitate delivery of education on lifestyle changes and therapy to all those at risk.
- A call and recall system from that register. This can be paper-based or electronic but must include patients unable to attend the practice. Agreement needs to be reached locally on how those most at need will be reviewed.
- A care plan, protocol or pathway describing the path the patient will take through the system and their involvement. Referral to specialist care and whether shared care will operate through the practice recall system should be considered.

Mary MacKinnon and Diabetes UK provide plans for the systematic review of people with diabetes, detailing the essential features of initial management, regular review and annual review.[4, 5] Control of blood pressure and lipids was discussed in Chapter 6.

MONITORING BLOOD GLUCOSE

We discussed self-monitoring of blood glucose concentration in Chapter 6 and learned about patients who did not understand why they were measuring their blood sugar. It is imperative to have in place a protocol that allows interpretation of these results for the patient and discussion around action to be taken. The National Institute for Health and Clinical Excellence (NICE) provided guidance[7] (Box 7.1) in 2002. A consensus statement was published in 2005, which is considered up to date[8] and provides a template for frequency of testing. and, in the full document, a useful algorithm.[6]

BOX 7.1   NICE guidance on blood glucose measurement

- Haemoglobin A_{1c} (HbA_{1c}) should be measured at intervals of 2–6 months. The appropriate interval for an individual patient should depend on:
  - acceptable levels of control, and
  - stability of blood glucose control, and/or
  - change in levels of blood glucose, and/or
  - change in therapies
- 6-monthly measurements should be made if the blood glucose level and blood glucose therapy are stable
- If measurement of HbA_{1c} is not possible because of abnormal erythrocyte turnover or haemoglobinopathy, use blood glucose profiles and/or total glycated haemoglobin estimation
- HbA_{1c} measurement should be DCCT aligned*

*Consistent with the system used in the Diabetes Control and Complications Trial.

CONTROLLING BLOOD GLUCOSE

Healthy eating, keeping active and maintaining an optimal weight are to be encouraged at every stage of diabetes. Remember type 2 diabetes is a progressive condition, and that to maintain blood glucose concentration at acceptable levels (Box 7.2) medication with hypoglycaemic agents or with insulin will often be required.

Oral hypoglycaemic agents

The oral hypoglycaemic agents available are set out in Table 7.1.

Insulin

People who have type 1 diabetes will always need to be treated with insulin until a successful method of restoring insulin output is found. Research is underway into inhaled insulin and

---

BOX 7.2   NICE targets for blood glucose control

- For each individual, a target HbA_{1c} (DCCT aligned) should be set between 6.5% and 7.5%, based on the risk of macrovascular and microvascular complications
- In general, the lower target HbA_{1c} is preferred for people at significant risk of macrovascular complications, but higher targets are necessary for those at risk of iatrogenic hypoglycaemia

---

TABLE 7.1   Oral hypoglycaemic agents for management of type 2 diabetes

Tablet	Name	Mode of action	Comments
Sulphonylureas	Examples: • glibenclamide • tolbutamide • gliclazide	Increase beta-cell insulin secretion. Often first-line choice in slim patients with type 2 disease, in whom beta-cell insulin output may be diminished	Longer acting agents, e.g. glibenclamide, are contraindicated in elderly patients. May cause episodes of hypoglycaemia ('hypos')
Postprandial glucose regulators	• repaglinide • nateglinide	Reduce blood glucose rise after meals through short, rapid action. Need to be taken at every meal	Fast-acting tablet taken before meals to regulate blood glucose. Can be added to metformin or taken alone. Less likely than sulphonylureas to cause hypos
Biguanides	• metformin	Decrease glucose output from liver and increase cellular response to insulin	Drug of first choice in overweight patients but may cause transient gastric disturbances; start at a low dose and titrate up
Thiazolidinediones	• rosiglitazone • pioglitazone	Improve insulin sensitivity. Can be used as monotherapy in overweight patients who cannot take metformin. *Recent NICE guidance was published before a change in the licence for thiazolidinediones*	Regular monitoring of liver function required. May cause oedema. Can be combined with above medications or used as monotherapy. Not licensed for combination with insulin
Alpha-glucosidase inhibitors	• acarbose	Reduces postprandial glucose peak by inhibiting gastrointestinal carbohydrate digestion	May cause initial gastric disturbances. Take care if using with sulphonylureas, because inhibition of glucose uptake makes glucose ineffective in the treatment of hypos

transplantation of insulin-secreting beta cells into other organs as alternatives to insulin injections.[7] People with type 2 diabetes may require insulin when oral medication is insufficient for the body's needs. Increasingly insulin is added to metformin or sulphonylureas in the management of type 2 diabetes.

Insulin types

Porcine insulin is chemically close to our own endogenous insulin and is considered less antigenic than bovine insulin. Synthetic 'human' insulins do not come from human sources but are produced by enzyme modification of porcine insulin or biosynthetically by DNA technology. They are even nearer chemically to endogenous insulin and therefore are less antigenic; they are cheaper to produce and widely available. Some people, when transferred from animal to human insulin, report losing their hypoglycaemia warning signs. When making this transfer, it is important to reduce the daily dosage and make adjustments in the light of home monitoring results. Insulins that are widely available are listed in Box 7.3, together with typical dosage regimens. It is not within the scope of this chapter to list all insulins; refer to the current edition of *MIMS*, which all GPs receive, for a useful chart and information on individual preparations. A patient's insulin regimen should be tailored to optimise their glucose control and to suit their lifestyle.

Insulin injectors

Choice of a suitable injector device requires consideration of various factors:

- Can the individual manage a refillable injector?
- Can he or she read the display?
- Does the device deliver the full dose required by the patient? Settings on pen injectors may go up in increments of one or two units, and range from 40 to 70 units.
- Is the device available on prescription?
- Does it take the type of insulin prescribed?

Liase with local diabetes specialist nurses until you are confident in the selection of insulin regimens and delivery devices.

Injection technique

One of the most common reasons for poor control of blood glucose is overuse of one site for insulin injections. This leads to formation of a pad of fatty tissue (lipohypertrophy) or destruction of tissue (lipodystrophy). This makes injections relatively painless, encouraging the site's repeated use, but adversely affects insulin absorption.[8] When assessing control, ask to see injection sites and advise site rotation.

SPECIAL GROUPS

We have focused on type 1 and type 2 diabetes, but it is important to maintain a high degree of suspicion in order to detect less common forms of diabetes.

Gestational diabetes

Diabetes can occur for the first time in pregnancy. Metabolic control should be tight, and if

BOX 7.3   Insulins for the management of type 1 and type 2 diabetes*

INSULIN	TYPICAL REGIMEN

Rapid-acting insulin analogue

- Modified form of human insulin
- Very rapid action – can be taken with meals
- Clear
- Onset: < 15 minutes
- Duration: 2–5 hours
- NovoRapid, Humalog, Apidra

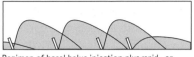

Regimen of basal bolus injection plus rapid- or short-acting insulin with each meal

Short-acting insulin

- Soluble
- Clear
- Onset: 30 minutes
- Peak: 1–3 hours
- Duration: ≤ 8 hours
- E.g. Actrapid, Humulin S, Hypurin Porcine or Bovine Neutral, Insuman Rapid

Basal bolus: once-daily injection of a medium- or long-acting insulin plus short- or rapid-acting insulin with each meal (e.g. Humulin I and Humalog, Human Monotard and Actrapid, Lantus and NovoRapid)

Medium- and long-acting insulin

- Crystals in suspension (need re-suspending)
- Cloudy
- NPH (Neutral Protamine Hagedorn) or Isophane
- Onset: 1.5 hours
- Peak: 4–12 hours
- Duration: ≤ 24 hours
- E.g. Human Insulatard, Humulin I, Hypurin Porcine or Isophane

Once-daily injection of medium- or long-acting insulin (e.g. Human Monotard, Humulin Lente, Lantus)

Premixed insulin

- Premixed combinations of short- and intermediate-acting insulins (biphasic)
- Cloudy (needs re-suspending)
- Different combinations of mix (e.g. 30/70 mixture = 30% fast-acting + 70% intermediate-acting)
- Onset: 30 minutes
- Peak: 2–8 hours
- Duration: ≤ 24 hours
- E.g. Mixtard 10, 20, etc.; Humulin M1, M2, etc.; Insuman Comb 15, 25, 50
- Also analogue mixtures, e.g. NovoMix 30, Humalog Mix 25

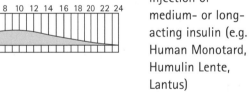

Twice-daily injection of an insulin mixture (e.g. Human Mixtard 30, Humulin M3)

Long-acting insulin

- Glargine (Lantus) and detemir (Levemir) are long-acting insulins which have an action of up to 24 hours but which do not have a distinct peak of action

*Based on information produced by Novo Nordisk. It is not within the scope of this article to list all insulins. The current edition of MIMS, which all GPs receive, has a useful chart and individual information

treatment is needed to control blood glucose it must be insulin. Any younger women with type 2 diabetes managed by oral hypoglycaemic agents and considering pregnancy should transfer to insulin as early as possible.

Women who have had gestational diabetes are more prone to diabetes in later life and should be advised accordingly. They should be offered regular screening for diabetes. Further information is available from Diabetes UK.[9]

Maturity-onset diabetes of the young (MODY)

This difficult-to-recognise inherited condition develops in young people, up to the age of 25 years. It is often treated with tablets, but insulin may be needed. Useful advice for patients can be found on the Diabetes UK website.[10]

Slow-onset type 1 diabetes in the elderly

Type 1 diabetes of slow onset is not a separate form of diabetes but should be suspected in an elderly patient with symptoms that do not respond to oral medication, especially if he or she is of slim to normal body build. When an individual's beta cells are failing to secrete insulin, muscle is metabolised to gain energy, leading to ketone formation and weight loss, and a high level of suspicion should be adopted for anyone with the following symptoms:

- weight loss – may be marked in people with normal or low body mass index (BMI)
- oliguria, frequency
- uncontrollable high blood glucose levels despite oral therapy
- increasing lethargy and malaise
- ketones in urine or blood (not always present if the condition is caught early).

Frequent review is required to confirm the diagnosis of slow-onset type 1 diabetes. Insulin is needed at an early stage.

DETECTING AND MANAGING COMPLICATIONS

Complications of diabetes can be categorised roughly into:

- microvascular – retinopathy, nephropathy and neuropathy (more likely in type 1 but do occur in type 2)
- macrovascular – cardiovascular disease, stroke and peripheral vascular disease (more likely in type 2).

If hypertension and erectile dysfunction were included, 65–70% of those with type 2 disease would have complications at diagnosis.[11]

A systematic approach to diabetes must include measures for the early detection of these damaging effects of diabetes. MacKinnon and Diabetes UK provide guidance that can be tailored to your needs, but some points need emphasis:

- Early detection of the 'at risk' foot requires assessment by a trained health professional and liaison with local podiatrists.[12]
- A key element of the NSF for Diabetes is the introduction of quality-controlled eye screening for all who have diabetes. NICE published guidance and primary care trusts (PCTs) will be putting this into practice by 2007.[13]
- Kidney disease can be detected early by testing the urine for microalbuminuria (the presence of microscopic amounts of protein undetectable by Albustix). There are several methods of screening and more than one result is needed to confirm the diagnosis (see the NICE website for guidance[14]).
- Men with diabetes may not disclose information about erectile dysfunction. A member of the diabetes care team with training in this sensitive area of care should broach the subject. UK Management Guidelines for Erectile Dysfunction are available online.[15]

We have discussed prevention of coronary heart disease (CHD) and diabetes emergencies, including hyperglycaemia, in Chapters 5 and 6.

ACTIVITY

Think about your practice: how do you help people with diabetes play their part in achieving good control of their diabetes?

Do you ask about erectile dysfunction? If not, who does?

HYPOGLYCAEMIC ATTACK

A 'hypo' or, to give it its full name, hypoglycaemic attack occurs when the blood glucose level drops too low. Diabetes UK suggests 4 mmol/l as a minimum blood-glucose level, hence their slogan 'Four is the Floor'.[6]

Hypos can be caused by sulphonylureas, which increase insulin secretion, or by insulin injections. Hypos induced by sulphonylureas (especially glibenclamide, which is long acting) may be protracted.

Hypos have been described as unavoidable.[16] And yet, along with fear of possible complications, they are the aspect of diabetes most feared by those who have to live with the disease.[17] People's concerns relate to fear of losing consciousness, of displaying inconsistent behaviour and of losing control or looking drunk. They may also worry about driving and the possibility of losing their licence.

It is not within the scope of this chapter to cover treatment options, but practice nurses would be well advised to acquaint themselves with the local guidelines on dealing with this emergency.

CONCLUSION

A systematic approach to the early detection of complications in people with diabetes is essential. Successful control of metabolism through lifestyle and medication is paramount. Type 2 diabetes is a progressive condition and medication will need to be continually reviewed and tailored to the individual. National guidance is available both for the health professional and the person with diabetes.

EVALUATION ACTIVITY

Considering your own practice, identify one area of diabetes management that you do well and one that you would like to improve.

Discuss with other team members how you would like to enhance patient care.

LEARNING POINTS

- There is a need for a call and recall system for everyone with diabetes
- Treatment for diabetes needs to be tailored to the individual patient and include lifestyle advice
- Women who develop gestational diabetes are prone to developing diabetes later in life
- Early screening measures can prevent or halt diabetic complications

REFERENCES

1. Department of Health. National Service Framework for Diabetes: Standards and Delivery Strategy. London: DoH, 2002. Available at: http://www.dh.gov.uk/PolicyAndGuidance/HealthAndSocialCareTopics/Diabetes/fs/en
2. DCCT Research Group. The effect of intensive treatment of diabetes on the development and progression of long-term complications in insulin-dependent diabetes mellitus. N Engl J Med 1993; 329: 977–986.
3. Gray A, Clarke P, Farmer A, Holman R. Implementing intensive control of blood glucose concentration and blood pressure in type 2 diabetes in England: cost analysis (UKPDS 63). BMJ 2002; 325: 860–863.
4. MacKinnon M. Providing Diabetes Care in General Practice. London: Class Publishing, 2002.
5. 5. Diabetes UK. Recommendations for the Provision of Services in Primary Care for People with

Diabetes. London: Diabetes UK, 2005. Available at: http://www.diabetes.org.uk/hcpreports/primary_recs.pdf

6. National Institute for Health and Clinical Excellence. Management of Type 2 Diabetes. Management of Blood Glucose. Inherited Guideline G. London: NICE, 2002. Available at: http://www.nice.org.uk

7. Owens D, Barnett AH, Pickup J, et al. The continuing debate on self-monitoring of blood glucose. Diabetes Primary Care 2005; 6(1): 9–21.

8. Jones EW. An Illustrated Guide for the Diabetic Clinic. London: Blackwell Science, 1998.

9. Diabetes UK. Recommendations for the Management of Pregnant Women with Diabetes (including Gestational Diabetes). London: Diabetes UK, 2005. Available at: http://www.diabetes.org.uk/infocentre/carerec/preg4.doc

10. Diabetes Q&A on MODY. Available at: http://www.diabetes.org.uk/infocentre/inform/mody.htm

11. Kings Fund Report. Counting the Cost . The Real Impact of Non Insulin Dependent Diabetes. London: Diabetes UK, 1996.

12. National Diabetes Support Team. Diabetic Foot Guide. 2006. Available at: http://www.diabetes.nhs.uk/downloads/NDST_Diabetic_Foot_Guide.pdf

13. National Institute for Health and Clinical Excellence. Management of Type 2 Diabetes. Retinopathy – Screening and Early Management. Inherited Clinical Guideline E. London: DoH, 2002. Available at: http://www.nice.org.uk

14. National Institute for Health and Clinical Excellence. Management of Type 2 Diabetes. Renal Disease – Prevention and Early Management. Inherited Guideline F. London: DoH, 2002. Available at: http://www.nice.org.uk

15. Ralph D, McNicholas T. UK management guidelines for erectile dysfunction. BMJ 2000; 321: 499–503.

16. Working Party Report. Diabetes & Cognitive Function: The Evidence So Far. London: BDA (now Diabetes UK), 1996.

17. Brian M, Frier. Morbidity of hypoglycaemia. Diabetes Rev International 1994; 3(2).

FURTHER INFORMATION

Campbell H, Hotchkiss R, Bradshaw N, Porteous M. Integrated care pathways. BMJ 1998; 316: 133–137. An informative article on integrated care pathways that could be adapted to diabetes.

Diabetes and Primary Care Journal: contact SB Communications: Tel. 0207 627 1510.

Diabetes UK: highlight examples of good practice. http://www.diabetes.org.uk/sharedpractice

National Institute for Health and Clinical Excellence: when considering what education strategies work for people with diabetes, try the guidance from NICE on the use of patient-education models for diabetes. Technology Appraisal 60. London: DoH, April 2003. Available at the NICE website: http://www.nice.org.uk/cat.asp?c=68326

Chapter 8

DIABETES
Promoting patient involvement

Gwen Hall

LEARNING OBJECTIVES

After reading this chapter you will be able to:

- discuss new ways of working through the new General Medical Services (GMS) Contract
- list the components of a patient-held record for a person with diabetes
- outline methods of empowering people with diabetes to participate in their own care
- devise a protocol for diabetes care based on participation by members of the primary care team, secondary care and people with diabetes

Chapters 5–7 have demonstrated that diabetes mellitus is a serious condition that needs to be managed systematically to prevent the development of complications. Type 1 disease (previously called insulin-dependent or juvenile-onset diabetes) is rapid in onset and requires life-long insulin injections. The much more frequent and increasingly common type 2 disease develops more insidiously and is managed by diet, activity and oral therapy and/or, increasingly, insulin. In both conditions, excellent control of blood glucose can delay or halt the microvascular complications of retinopathy and nephropathy.

In type 2 disease, macrovascular complications are more significant and blood pressure control is vitally important in the prevention of coronary heart disease (CHD), peripheral vascular disease and stroke. Targets for blood pressure and blood lipid and glucose levels have been set, and in this chapter we address the teamwork required to meet them, empowering the person with diabetes to participate in that process.[1–3]

The new contract for the provision of general medical services (GMS) by general practice teams also sets targets relating to the management in primary care of long-term conditions such as diabetes.

The importance of patient participation is increasingly recognised, and people with diabetes can become involved in the management of their condition at several levels:

- receiving one-to-one education from a trained practice nurse
- as an 'expert patient'
- working with a primary care trust (PCT) as a 'diabetes champion'.

These will be discussed in turn, with advice on agreeing protocols and cementing links with secondary care.

THE NEW GMS CONTRACT

On 20 June 2003 GPs accepted the new GMS Contract that was implemented in April 2004 and updated in 2006.[4] The new Contract:

- has increased funding in primary care
- encourages new ways of working within primary care teams
- rewards practices (rather than individual GPs) for delivering higher levels of care – points are awarded according to a quality and outcomes framework designed to promote good chronic disease management (Table 8.1)
- supports new measures to ensure patient choice and access to a wider range of high-quality services, with more treatment in the community and less in hospitals
- provides new career opportunities for practice nurses.

Booklets are available that explain how practices can meet the quality targets and detail opportunities for primary care in the new Contract.[4] The key role of practice nurses in systematic chronic disease management has been recognised by the Department of Health (DoH), and many of the Contract's key quality indicators (Table 8.1) relate to diabetes. The full list is available at the DoH website.[5]

TABLE 8.1 The GMS Contract (2006) sets targets for chronic disease management	
Hitting the targets earns the practice points and thus increases its income	
Disease area	Points available
Secondary prevention of coronary heart disease*	89
Heart failure*	20
Stroke or transient ischaemic attacks (TIAs)*	24
Hypertension*	83
Diabetes*	93
Chronic obstructive pulmonary disease (COPD)	33
Epilepsy	15
Hypothyroidism	7
Cancer	11
Palliative care	6
Mental health	39
Asthma	45
Dementia	20
Depression*	33
Chronic kidney disease*	27
Atrial fibrillation*	30
Obesity*	8
Learning disabilities	4
Smoking indicators	68
Total points for achieving clinical standards	655
*Possibly diabetes related.	

NSF DELIVERY STRATEGY

In the National Service Framework (NSF) for Diabetes: Delivery Strategy, the DoH firmly places the patient at the centre of care.

In order to achieve the targets set for diabetes care, people with the condition should have a personal diabetes record that contains:[5]

- the clinical record of care
- current and past treatment regimens
- results of investigations
- a management plan with agreed goals and targets
- a local contact for advice.

Remember that people with diabetes provide their own day-to-day care. They must be given the tools to do the job. Long-term management of diabetes was discussed in Chapter 7.

ACTIVITY

Thinking of your own practice, do you provide people with diabetes with a personal record?

Do all members of the team contribute?

Does it fit into shared care with specialists?

EDUCATION, SELF-CARE AND PATIENT-CENTRED CARE

By undertaking this learning exercise you have shown an interest in continuing your education. The latest (2004) edition of the Nursing and Midwifery Council (NMC) *Code of Professional Conduct* incorporates guidance on enlarging the scope of a nurse's practice.[6] This places a specific requirement on the nurse to maintain professional skills and competencies:

If an aspect of practice is beyond your level of competence you must obtain help and supervision from a competent practitioner until you and your employer consider that you have acquired the requisite knowledge and skill.

Nurses are being encouraged to develop a 'specialist interest' in various fields and must have the training to enable them to do so. Methods of ensuring this training is effective are described in the DoH publication *Liberating the Talents*:[7]

- Practical training, which could be provided by a GP, consultant or other nurse, will enable the nurse to acquire new skills. Think about using clinical skills laboratories if available. Ensure that both learner and educator have clear expectations about the learning outcomes and standards required from skills training.
- Establish a mechanism for documenting that practitioners have achieved required standards and ensure nurses record attainment of competence in their professional development portfolios.
- Multidisciplinary training may be the best way of developing skills and knowledge and building the team at the same time.
- Regular clinical supervision will enable the assessment of achievement and maintenance of competence.

This enthusiasm for learning needs to be fostered in patients and their carers also. There is emerging evidence that group education is effective and is a way of promoting self-care through contact with others and sharing ideas.

People deserving of special attention for diabetes education include the elderly infirm, those with learning difficulties and those for whom English is not their first language.[8]

ACTIVITY

What are the barriers to learning for your patients with diabetes?

How can your team enhance your systems of education?

EXPERT PATIENTS

Health professionals need to consider ways in which people with diabetes can be actively engaged in their own care and education. In 1999 the Chief Medical Officer set up the Expert Patients Task Force, to consider ways of involving lay people in chronic disease management. The task force recommended the introduction of lay-led self-management training programmes, with pilot sites to be phased in over the following years. These programmes are becoming more readily available and are being evaluated.[9]

Eight further specific recommendations were:

- patient expertise to be utilised in formulating any care pathway for people with chronic disease
- more self-management courses for people with chronic disease to be established
- barriers to patient participation in these programmes, and their own care, are to be identified and methods of overcoming them sought
- patient-led self-management to be integrated into future NHS initiatives
- primary care trusts to arrange for delivery or commissioning of lay-led self-management programmes for key chronic conditions
- patient-led programmes to receive extra support in partnership with health and social care professionals
- build a core course that would promote health professionals' knowledge and understanding about the benefits, for them and for patients, of user-led self-management programmes
- establish a national coordinating and training resource to enable health, social services and

voluntary sector professionals to keep up to date with developments in the provision of self-management; patients should be part of the process of developing professional education programmes.

PROTOCOLS AND CARE PATHWAYS

Protocols and pathways help to clarify the role of health professionals and people with diabetes in providing systematic care. Who does what will depend on local circumstances, but a clear pathway from diagnosis to long-term care is required, stating the key elements and when they should occur in the programme. An example is shown in Figure 8.1.

The whole practice diabetes team should take part in deciding on a protocol, together with other health professionals such as dietitian and podiatrist, diabetes specialists and people with diabetes.[10] The process of agreeing a protocol need not be lengthy and could be based on published guidance (Figure 8.2).[11]

BUILDING BRIDGES

A good, locally agreed protocol will help build bridges between primary and secondary care. Primary care is taking more responsibility for diabetes, particularly type 2, and handling more of the systematic call and recall of all those on diabetes registers. This is being encouraged by the NSF and by the GMS Contract. It is important to agree referral policies for secondary care and to recognise when specialist input is desirable. Your PCT diabetes lead is a valuable contact; you might like to make contact with him or her and discuss local diabetes services.

As discussed in Chapter 7, the NSF for diabetes highlighted the need for champions in diabetes, both clinical and lay people. In general, champions are individuals who have a desire to improve

---

ACTIVITY

What opportunities exist locally for people with diabetes to join in structured programmes of education such as Expert Patient schemes?

How could you involve them in the management of diabetes within your practice?

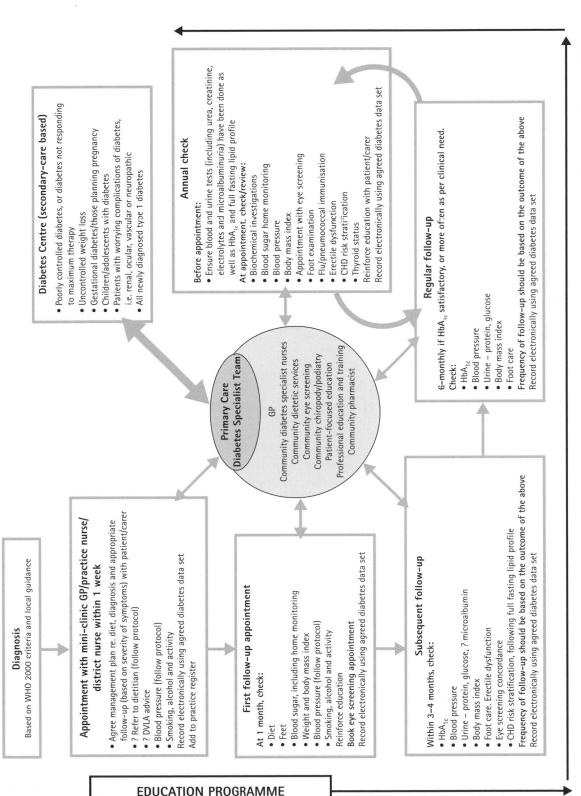

Figure 8.1   Diabetes integrated care pathway – an example of a protocol for diabetes care. (Courtesy of D. Russell-Jones and Guildford & Waverley PCT.)

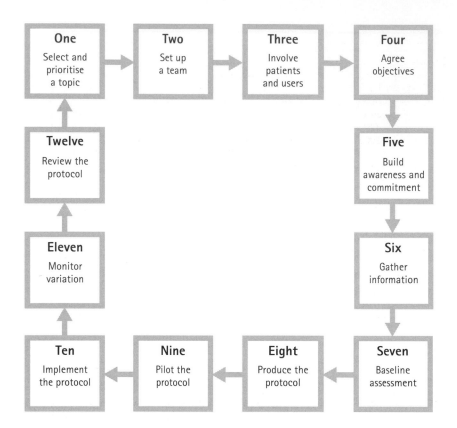

Figure 8.2 An approach to protocol development suggested by the NHS Modernisation Agency.[12]

services for people with a particular condition through working together, pooling their expertise and standing up for the needs of everyone who has a role in providing the necessary care.

CONCLUSION

The NSF for diabetes has highlighted the need for patient involvement in the delivery of high-quality diabetes care, while the new GMS Contract has provided the impetus for primary care to meet set targets in chronic disease management.

Expert patient programmes enable people with chronic disease to become effective participants in the education process and in mutual support. Practice nurses can be in the vanguard of agreeing protocols or pathways to streamline service delivery. By truly working together we can improve the quality of life for people with diabetes.

EVALUATION ACTIVITY

Considering your own practice, identify an area of patient involvement that you would like to improve.

Discuss how you would like to address this with members of your diabetes team.

LEARNING POINTS

- Effective diabetes care requires an agreed team approach
- The person with diabetes should be at the centre of their care
- Care pathways and protocols ensure cohesion in the delivery of high-quality care
- Practice nurses are in the vanguard of implementing the new GMS Contract

REFERENCES

1. National Institute for Health and Clinical Excellence. Management of Type 2 Diabetes. Management of Blood Pressure and Blood Lipids. Inherited Guideline H. London: NICE, 2002. Available at: http://www.nice.org.uk

2. National Institute for Health and Clinical Excellence. Management of Type 2 Diabetes. Management of Blood Glucose. Inherited Guideline G. London: NICE, 2002. Available at: http://www.nice.org.uk

3. Joint British Societies. Guidelines on prevention of cardiovascular disease in clinical practice. Heart 2005; 91: 1–52.

4. British Medical Association. General Medical Services Contract. London: BMA, 2006. Available at: http://www.bma.org.uk/ap.nsf/Content/Hubthenewgmscontract

5. Department of Health. National Service Framework for Diabetes: Delivery Strategy. London: DoH, 2002. Available at: http://www.dh.gov.uk/PolicyAndGuidance/HealthAndSocialCareTopics/Diabetes/fs/en

6. Nursing & Midwifery Council. Code of Professional Conduct 2002. Available at: http://www.nmc-uk.org/aFramedisplay.aspx?documentID=201

7. Department of Health. Liberating the Talents. April 2003. Available at: http://www.dh.gov.uk

8. National Institute for Health and Clinical Excellence. Guidance on the Use of Patient-education Models for Diabetes. Technology Appraisal 60. London: DoH, April 2003.

9. Department of Health. The Expert Patient. A New Approach to Chronic Disease Management for the 21st Century. London: DoH, 2001. Available at: http://www.expertpatients.nhs.uk

10. Diabetes UK. Recommendations for the Provision of Services in Primary Care for People with Diabetes. London: Diabetes UK. Available at: http://www.diabetes.org.uk

11. NHS Modernisation Agency. Protocol-based Care. A Step by Step Guide to Developing Protocols. Available at: http://www.modern.nhs.uk/protocolbasedcare

FURTHER INFORMATION

Department of Health: the NSFs for Older People and CHD are highly relevant to your diabetes practice. Both are available at: http://www.dh.gov.uk

NHS Confederation: *The Role of Nurses under the New GMS Contract*. This guidance for nurses was published when the first new GMS Contract was agreed. Although dated it does provide useful information on how nurses can work within the Contract. The role of nurses under the new GMS Contract. Available at: http://www.nhsconfed.org/docs/gmsbriefing7.pdf

NHS Modernisation Agency: *A Guide to Role Redesign in Diabetes Care*. Available from: NHS Modernisation Agency, Richmond House, 79 Whitehall, London SW1A 2NS; http://www.dh.gov.uk/assetRoot/04/06/74/11/04067411.pdf

NHS Modernisation Agency: *Protocol-based Care. A Step-by-step Guide to Developing Protocols*. A useful step-by-step guide for those who are new to writing protocols. Available at: http://www.modern.nhs.uk/protocolbasedcare

Chapter 9

MENTAL HEALTH
Recognising depression

Alyson Buck

LEARNING OBJECTIVES

After reading this chapter you will be able to:

- discuss the incidence of depression
- outline common signs and symptoms of depression
- have an understanding of the main treatment strategies for depressed individuals
- know when to refer a patient on to specialist services

In the National Service Framework (NSF) for Mental Health, published in 1999, the Government stated that mental health care would have 'the same priority as coronary heart disease'.[1] The NHS Plan and the Mental Health Policy Implementation Guide have built on this to ensure that mental health stays at the top of the healthcare agenda.[2,3]

In 1987, an estimated one-quarter of general practice consultations were for mental health problems.[4] The NHS Plan suggested that up to 50% of consultations are related to psychological

ACTIVITY

Obtain for your practice a copy of the National Service Framework for Mental Health.

Read through it to identify which aspects of your work relate to the seven identified targets.

distress, and that severe mental illness is more commonly managed by a primary care team than in secondary care.[2, 5]

The primary care team's responsibility for identification, assessment, management and prevention of common mental health problems, such as depression and anxiety, is affirmed in the NSF and the report to the Workforce Action Team of the Primary Care Key Group.[6]

The focus in this chapter is on depression.

EPIDEMIOLOGY

Depression is the most common mental health problem and the third most common reason for people to consult their GP.[7] Around one person in five is currently depressed, and up to one in three will experience depression at some point.[7]

It has serious effects on the physical health of those with the condition, and prevents many people from fulfilling their potential or playing an active part in everyday life.[8, 9] It is far from a trivial condition. The risk of suicide among depressed individuals is high.

In the UK, rates of depression are greatly influenced by age, sex, marital status and ethnicity. Up to the age of 55 years, almost twice as many women as men are affected, but after that the trend reverses. In people aged over 65 years depression is the most common mental health problem, with about 10–15% having significant depressive symptoms. The rate of depression is highest in widowed males, divorced females and those who have separated from a relationship. It is higher in single parents than couples and higher in couples with children than those without.[10, 11]

Data based on a relatively small sample of ethnic minority groups suggest that the depression rate among men corresponds to that for white males. However, the rate is higher among Asian and Oriental women than white women, and lower among West Indian and African women than white women.[10]

Unemployed women have more than twice the prevalence of depression than unemployed men, and major depression is strongly associated with circumstances such as poor housing or homelessness, and adverse events such as loss and bereavement.[12]

Worldwide, depression is predicted to be the second most common cause of morbidity by 2020. Several reports recommend locally agreed standards of practice and service delivery in mental health care, and many primary care trusts have protocols in place for the management of depression.[1, 3, 13, 14]

ACTIVITY

Review the profile of the patients registered with your practice. How many of them fall into the 'at risk' groups as identified above?

Consider why depression might be more common among these individuals.

Review your practice protocol on recognition of depression. If you do not have such a protocol, consider what should go in one.

SYMPTOMS OF DEPRESSION

Depressed mood is usually the main feature of depression, but other symptoms are common. Patients will visit the practice for a variety of reasons in the hope that the practice nurse or GP will recognise they are not coping well with life. An important service that the practice nurse can perform is to try to understand the patient's situation. What does having depression mean for them and their family? How deep is the hopelessness and despair that they feel?

Diagnostic criteria for major depressive disorder are outlined in Box 9.1, and five symptom domains that can be helpful in the recognition of depression in Box 9.2.

Assessment/screening for depression

If you suspect someone has depression, a comprehensive assessment (Box 9.3) is the first step. Because this is a 'whole-body' illness, this assessment should be holistic and observing and listening to the person takes skill. There are screening tools that can help confirm the diagnosis (see Box 9.4 and Further Information) but remember that these questionnaires are only a tool. Nothing can replace an objective, face-to-face assessment by an experienced nurse. Experience combined with appropriate tools should ensure prompt referral, to the GP or specialist services, where necessary.

BOX 9.1   Diagnostic criteria for major depressive disorder[15]

Five or more (during the previous 2 weeks) of the following:

- Depressed most of the day, for most days, indicated by subjective report or observation
- Diminished interest in (almost) all activities most of the day, nearly every day
- Weight loss or weight gain (±5%)
- Insomnia or hypersomnia
- Psychomotor agitation or retardation nearly every day (observed by others)
- Fatigue or loss of energy
- Feelings of unworthiness or excessive or inappropriate guilt
- Diminished ability to think or concentrate
- Recurrent thoughts of death, recurrent suicidal ideation

ACTIVITY

Referring to Boxes 9.1 and 9.2, reflect on the patients you see in your practice. How many of these might be depressed and not experiencing only a physical problem?

Consider the signs and symptoms they experience and/or present with.

Think of the worst day you have had, when you wondered 'What's the point?'. Now magnify those feelings 100 times, and reflect on the effect that might have on you and all aspects of your life. Now you are beginning to understand the impact depression has on an individual.

BOX 9.2   Five symptom domains in depression[16]

1. Physical symptoms
- Significant changes in bodily symptoms, generally reflecting a 'slowing down', e.g. reduced energy and poor appetite. Sometimes there is increased appetite and subsequent weight gain, increased agitation and physiological anxiety symptoms

2. Behaviour
- Avoidance of activities and withdrawal from social situations (perhaps reported as 'sitting around doing nothing', 'staying in bed all day'); stooped posture; avoidance of eye contact; monotonous and monosyllabic speech; self-neglect (poor personal hygiene)

3. Cognition (thought)
- Reduced concentration and impaired memory
- Possible expression of suicidal ideas
- Negative thinking style, centring around:
  - the self: 'I can't do anything', 'I'm no good at that'
  - the world and other people: 'Other people don't like me', 'They all think I'm no good', 'The world's a horrible place'
  - the future: 'The future's bleak', 'I'll never get better', 'Things will never improve'

4. Affect (mood)
- Low mood, poor motivation; 'I don't feel like doing anything', 'I feel flat' and 'I can't enjoy anything'

5. Environment
- Changed social circumstances, e.g. loss of a loved one, redundancy, prolonged periods of anxiety

BOX 9.3   Information needed for assessment
Biographical Name, address, age, occupation
Biological Temperature, pulse, respiration, blood pressure, height; changes in appetite, weight, sleep pattern and libido
Psychological The patient's description of problems/symptoms; mood level, anxiety, suicidal/self-harm thoughts; thought content/disturbance; concerns about health/well-being; acts of deliberate self-harm; recent accidents
Social Changes in employment, relationships, hobbies/interests; use of alcohol/drugs (increasing consumption)

BOX 9.4   Screening tools for depression
General Health Questionnaire 12 questions for use with adults aged 16–74 years; takes 2–3 minutes to complete
Beck Depression Inventory Assesses severity of a depressive illness and measures change over time; for patients with more severe depression. The original version has 21 questions; the shorter 13-question version takes about 3 minutes to fill in
Edinburgh Postnatal Depression Scale Used where depression after childbirth is suspected, and also more widely to screen for antenatal depression. The 10-item self-report questionnaire is quick and easy to complete and acceptable to most women
Geriatric Depression Scale 15 questions; takes 3–4 minutes to complete
Hospital and Anxiety Depression Scale 14 questions; devised to detect and monitor anxiety and depression

TREATMENT OPTIONS

Most people with depression will be managed in primary care, but adequate pathways of care and collaborative working practices need to evolve. The NHS Plan emphasises new ways of communication between primary care and secondary/specialist care services.[2]

Well-informed practice nurses can educate, encourage and support depressed patients in appropriate use of medication. Many patients value the opportunity to talk in confidence to a non-judgemental person. The practice nurse can guide them towards community psychiatric nurses (CPNs), mental health social workers, psychologists, psychiatrists, day-care services and support groups. Depression can be effectively managed using a variety of therapeutic approaches.

ACTIVITY
Consider a patient that you thought about for the previous activity:
How was this person assessed? Were all the domains outlined in Box 9.2 included?
If not, can you identify any changes to your assessment protocol for improving the recognition of depression?
How might depression be affecting their ability to carry out routine activities?
Are they functioning effectively at work?
Are relationships with family and friends affected?

Pharmacological interventions

Drug treatment is usually with antidepressant medication, although anxiolytic drugs may also be used. Tricyclic antidepressants (TCAs) are used widely and are effective.

Selective serotonin reuptake inhibitors (SSRIs) are also used extensively; there seems no evidence that these are more effective than TCAs, but the different side-effect profile means they are often better tolerated. Sedation seems less of a problem with SSRIs, which is important for those patients who continue to work or drive. In addition it seems that SSRIs are less cardiotoxic in over-dosage, and are therefore preferred where there is a significant risk of deliberate self-harm.[17]

Monoamine oxidase inhibitors (MAOIs) tend not to be used as a first-line treatment as there are dangerous interactions with some foods and they may also be less effective than TCAs and SSRIs. Newer antidepressants – serotonin and noradren-aline reuptake inhibitors (SNRIs) such as fluox-etine (Prozac) and paroxetine (Seroxat) – are commonly used, and newer still are SNRIs such as venlafaxine (Efexor) and mirtazapine (Zispin), with the most recent addition being escitalopram (Cipralex).

Seroxat has been in the news in recent years because of court action against the manufacturers. Guidelines from the Committee on Safety of Medicines (CSM) state it should not be used in patients under 18 years old (see Further Inform-ation). Whatever antidepressant drug the patient is on, practice nurses need to reinforce that:

- antidepressants are not addictive but with-drawal needs to be managed carefully – abrupt withdrawal may lead to symptoms similar to those experienced prior to treatment
- patients need to give their treatment time to work (at least 4 weeks)
- treatment will probably need to continue for 4–6 months after recovery to prevent relapse.[18]

Psychosocial interventions

Evaluation has shown the benefit of approaches such as cognitive–behaviour therapy, behavioural activation, counselling, solution-focused brief therapy, etc., in depression. They work by identi-fying and challenging the thoughts and behaviour patterns adopted by the individual to cope with their feelings.

Behavioural activation explores the nature, essence and meaning of the depressive episode, and how the patient uses avoidance behaviour to cope with it.

Cognitive–behaviour therapy exposes patterns of thinking that may cause features of depression, and helps people to weaken connections between troublesome situations and habitual reactions to them.

Solution-focused brief therapy aims to build on solutions rather than focus on the problems a patient might have. Goals are set, and ways found to use a patient's own strengths and unique resources to accomplish them by exploring exceptions (periods when the patient does not experience the problems) and instances (periods when the patient experiences the problems, in whole or in part).

Complementary therapies

Therapeutic touch and massage with certain aromatherapy oils have been used with a degree of efficacy.[19] St. John's wort (*Hypericum perforatum*) is used worldwide as a homeopathic treatment for mild-to-moderate depression, and is better toler-ated and has fewer side-effects than many anti-depressant drugs.[20, 21] However, it interacts with conventional drugs such as certain contraceptives, antiepileptic drugs and other antidepressants, so patients must be advised accordingly.[17]

The effectiveness of taking omega-3 supple-ments (found in fish oils) in preventing depress-ion is being researched.[22]

Electroconvulsive therapy

Although controversial, electroconvulsive therapy (ECT) is still used, typically for severe depression. It is generally used only after other treatments have proved ineffective. ECT is thought to increase the level of neurotransmitters in the brain.[23]

ACTIVITY

Select two of the treatment options mentioned and find out more about them through further reading.

Find out where your local mental health team is based, and identify the community practice nurse who links with your practice.

RELAPSE PREVENTION

'Relapse' occurs when symptoms return within 6 months of apparent recovery, while 'recurrence' denotes their return after 6 months or longer free of symptoms.[24] Some surveys suggest that the total duration of a depressive episode is 6–9 months, although some last much longer. Many of the non-pharmacological interventions mentioned are useful in relapse prevention and might be used on a longer term basis. Drug therapy can also protect against relapse and may need to be used for up to 6 months after recovery.

Depression can be cyclical, recurring at certain times of the year or under certain circumstances in affected individuals. Developing a close relationship with a patient and keeping in regular contact with them will help the nurse to identify individual patterns and signs of relapse. Some

---

EVALUATION ACTIVITY

Reflect on the current care of clients with a long-term condition in your area.

Have they been screened for depression?

What are the strengths and weaknesses of your clinical care?

---

doctors believe it may be advantageous to increase antidepressant medication at times of expected recurrence, as a prophylactic measure. Regular communication with any specialist services involved in the patient's care is also essential.

CONCLUSION

Depression is a complex condition with no single cause. It varies in severity and duration and can have a marked effect on the health of the individual's family and on their work and social relationships. It is common and, because it is underdetected and undertreated, causes extended suffering for individuals and their families and carers. There is effective treatment, in a variety of forms, that can treat the depressive episode and prevent relapse. Most patients will be treated in primary care. Practice nurses are therefore ideally placed to work with them and their families, and should also aim to forge closer collaborative working practices with others who play a part in the patients' care.

LEARNING POINTS

- Depression is predicted to be the second most common cause of morbidity by 2020
- A comprehensive assessment is the first step in identifying depression
- Managegement is best approached by a combination of therapeutic and psychopharmacological interventions
- Most people with depression are managed in primary care
- Well-informed practice nurses are ideally placed to support depressed people

---

REFERENCES

1. Department of Health. National Service Framework for Mental Health. London: The Stationery Office, 1999.

2. Department of Health. The NHS Plan: A Plan for Investment A Plan for Reform. London: The

Stationery Office, 2000.

3. Department of Health. Mental Health Policy Implementation Guide. London: The Stationery Office, 2001.

4. Goldberg D, Bridges K. Screening for psychiatric illness in general practice: the general practitioner versus the screening questionnaire. J R Coll Gen Pract 1987; 37: 15–18.

5. Newell R, Gournay K. Mental Health Nursing – An Evidence Based Approach. London: Churchill Livingstone, 2000.

6. Department of Health. Workforce Action Teams: Primary Care Key Group Report to the WAT. London: DoH, 2001.

7. Improving the recognition and management of depression in primary care. Effect Health Care Bull 2002; 7(5): 9.

8. Murray CJ, Lopez AD. Alternative projections of mortality and disability by cause 1990–2020: global burden of disease study. Lancet 1997; 349: 1498–1504.

9. Jonsson B, Bebbington P. Economic studies of the treatment of depressive illness. In: Jonsson B, Bebbington P (eds), Health Economics of Depression. Chichester: Wiley, 1993.

10. Dinan T. The physical consequences of depressive illness. BMJ 1999; 318: 826–827.

11. Meltzer H, Gill B, Petticrew M, Hinds K. Economic activity and social functioning of adults with psychiatric disorders. OPCS Survey of Psychiatric Morbidity, Report 3. London: HMSO, 1995.

12. Gill B, Meltzer H, Hinds K. The prevalence of psychiatric morbidity among homeless adults. Economic activity and social functioning of adults with psychiatric disorders. OPCS Survey of Psychiatric Morbidity, Report 3. London: HMSO, 1996.

13. Clinical Standards Advisory Group. Services for Patients with Depression. London: Department of Health, 1999.

14. National Institute for Health and Clinical Excellence. Management of Depression in Primary and Secondary Care. Draft for 2nd Consultation, 2004. Available at: http://www.nice.org.uk

15. American Psychiatric Association (APA). Diagnostic & Statistical Manual of Mental Disorders, 4th edn, text revision. Washington, DC: APA, 2000.

16. Greenberger D, Padesky CA. Mind Over Mood: Changing the Way you Feel by Changing the Way you Think. New York: Guildford Press, 1995.

17. British Medical Association, The Royal Pharmaceutical Society of Great Britain. British National Formulary. London: BMA/RPSGB, 2006.

18. Blenkiron P. The management of depression in primary care: a summary of evidence-based guidelines. Psychiat Care 1998; 5: 172–177.

19. Field T. Touch Therapy. London: Churchill Livingstone, 2000.

20. Harrer G, Hubner WD, Podzuweit H. Effectiveness and tolerance of the hypericum extract LI 160 compared to maprotiline: a multi-centre double-blind study. J Geriat Psychiat Neurol 1994; 7(Suppl 1): S24–S28.

21. Linde K, Ramirez G, Mulrow CD, et al. St. John's wort for depression: an overview and meta-analysis of randomised clinical trials. BMJ 1996; 313: 253–258.

22. Severus WE, Littman AB, Stoll AL. Omega-3 fatty acids, homocysteine, and the increased risk of cardiovascular mortality in major depressive disorder. Harv Rev Psychiatry 2001; 9(6): 280–293.

23. Morrison-Valfre M. Foundations of Mental Health Care, 2nd edn. London: Mosby, 2001.

24. Bond AJ, Lader MH. Understanding Drug Treatment in Mental Health Care. Chichester: Wiley, 1996.

FURTHER INFORMATION

NICE. Depression: The Management of Depression in Primary and Secondary Care. Guideline. 6 December 2004. Available at: http://www.nice.org.uk

Screening tools

Beck A, Ward CH, Mendelssohn M, Erbaugh J. An inventory for measuring depression. Arch Gen Psychiatry 1961; 4: 561–571.

Cox JL, Holden JM, Sagovsky R. Detection of postnatal depression: development of the 10-item Edinburgh Postnatal Scale. Br J Psychiatry 1987; 150: 782–786.

Goldberg D. A User's Guide to the General Health Questionnaire. Windsor: NFER-Nelson. Available at: http://www.nfer-nelson.co.uk

Yesavage JA, Brink TL, Rose TL, et al. Development and validation of a geriatric depression screening scale: a preliminary report. J Psychiat Res 1983; 17: 37–49.

Zigmond AS, Snaith RP. The Hospital Anxiety and Depression Scale. Acta Psychiat Scand 1983; 67: 361–370.

Chapter 10

MENTAL HEALTH
Diagnosis of dementia

Alyson Buck

CHAPTER CONTENTS

LEARNING OBJECTIVES

After reading this chapter you will be able to:

- outline some of the different types of dementia
- identify common differential diagnoses of dementia
- distinguish the symptoms of dementia from depression and acute confusion

There is mounting evidence that early recognition and treatment of dementia can facilitate effective treatment by delaying cognitive decline and maintaining functioning.[1-3] Practice nurses are regularly in contact with people with dementia, as many will have physical health problems or disabilities. In addition, carers are likely to contact the practice nurse about their own health problems or difficulties associated with their relative's behaviour or decline.

The Audit Commission reported in 2002 that GPs need more support in the care of this patient group. Two-fifths were reluctant to diagnose dementia early, most did not use protocols to help diagnose dementia or depression, more than one-third felt they lacked ready access to specialist advice and just under half felt they had not received sufficient training for dementia.[3] The authors of a 2003 study conclude that 'all community-based nurses should be able to recognize the possibility of dementia and support those undergoing referral or assessment.' They go on to state that:

> Training in dementia recognition, and involvement in and membership of primary care teams supporting people with dementia should not be confined to community mental health nurses (CMHNs). All nurses who regularly encounter the general population of older people may be well placed to provide continuity of support for those who may, or may not, have cause to suspect that they or their relatives have early dementia.[4]

EPIDEMIOLOGY

The National Service Framework for Older People (NSFOP; Standard 7: Mental Health in Older People) estimates that, of the population aged over 65 years, about 5% have dementia, and at any one time 10–15% will have depression.[1] The National Institute for Health and Clinical Excellence (NICE) believes that as many as 700,000 people have dementia, the cause in 400,000 being Alzheimer's disease. Of those with mild to moderate Alzheimer's disease 15,000 will be under 70 years old, 75,000 will be 70–80 years old and 160,000 will be over 80 years old.[5]

The 3% or so under 65 years of age experience disproportionately high morbidity and more dramatic social consequences. Around 80% of people with dementia live at home, and 23% of these live alone. A GP with 1,500–2,000 patients can expect 12–20 of these to have a dementia.

Dementia seems to affect all groups in society equally, with no apparent link to gender, social class, ethnic group or geographical location.

WHAT IS DEMENTIA?

'Dementia is a term used to describe various brain disorders that have in common loss of brain function which is usually progressive and eventually severe'.[6] Alzheimer's disease is only one of more than 100 types of dementia (Box 10.1). Dementia damages short-term memory; affected individuals consistently forget things they have just said or done but can recall clearly events from years ago, often in great detail. They eventually lose their sense of time and place, and find it difficult to learn new information and do new things. As the disease progresses, help is needed with even the most basic functions of everyday living and behavioural problems may occur. Most eventually become uncommunicative and incontinent, and need 24-hour care. The time span for progression varies from 2 years to as many as 15–20 years, and dementia is not usually the cause of death.

DIFFERENTIAL DIAGNOSIS

Numerous conditions can cause a decline in cognitive function and dementia should not be diagnosed too readily.[7] The most important differential diagnoses are depression and acute confusional state (Table 10.1).

ACTIVITY

Obtain copies of the National Service Framework for Older People[1] and the Audit Commission's report Forget me Not[3] from the relevant websites.

Read these to establish what the priorities are in relation to the mental health of older people.

ACTIVITY

Consider the information in Box 10.1. Find out more about types of dementia unfamiliar to you, particularly those that are likely to be more common in your patient group (e.g. Alzheimer's disease, vascular dementia and Lewy-body dementia).

BOX 10.1   The more common types of dementia*

Alzheimer's disease
- Accounts for about half of all cases
- Deposits (or plaques) of an abnormal protein are found throughout the brain, and tangles of twisted protein molecules in the brain's nerve cells
- Scans detect atrophy of the cerebral cortex and widespread death of brain cells

Vascular (multi-infarct) dementia
- Brain damage is caused by tiny strokes arising from insufficient blood supply to the brain

Lewy-body dementia
- Regarded by some as a variant of Alzheimer's disease
- Proteins build up in the nerve cells of the brain

Frontotemporal dementia
- For example, Pick's disease
- Similarities to Alzheimer's disease, but many differences
- Striking changes in behaviour precede memory problems
- Onset typically in the 40s or 50s
- Marked inability to express oneself through speech

Huntington's disease (Huntington's chorea)
- Relatively rare inherited disorder
- Manifests itself in middle age, with jerky movements in addition to progressive dementia

AIDS-related dementia
- Most HIV-positive people will not experience dementia, but many who progress to AIDS will develop a severe dementia
- The cause may be HIV virus in the brain, or tumours or infections resulting from reduced immunity

Creutzfeldt–Jakob disease (CJD)
- 'Original' CJD usually occurs in middle age
- 'New variant CJD' (vCJD) occurs in younger people and progresses rapidly, often to death within 1 year
- There has been much publicity about the link between vCJD and eating beef from cattle infected with bovine spongiform encephalopathy (BSE)

Other
- Dementia can also result from excessive use of alcohol, brain tumours (e.g. meningioma), Parkinson's disease (occurs in 10–20%), normal pressure hydrocephalus and treatable causes, such as hormone and vitamin deficiencies, endocrine disturbances and infections (e.g. neurosyphilis).

*Adapted from Cayton et al.[6]

Acute confusional state

Acute confusion usually develops over hours or days, most often as a result of infection (particularly of the urinary or respiratory tract) or drug toxicity. There are usually signs of physical ill health.

It is important to check any medication that has been taken (or omitted). All symptoms resolve with treatment of the underlying cause.

TABLE 10.1   Clinical features of dementia, depression and acute confusional state[7]

Feature	Dementia	Acute confusional state	Depression
Onset	Insidious	Acute	Gradual
Duration	Months/years	Hours/days	Weeks/months
Course	Stable and progressive. Vascular dementia usually stepwise and fluctuating (worse at night)	Lucid periods, usually worse in mornings	Improves as the day goes on
Alertness	Usually normal	Fluctuates	Normal
Orientation	May be normal: usually impaired for time/place	Always impaired: time/place/person	Usually normal
Memory	Impaired recent and sometimes remote memory	Recent impaired	Recent may be impaired, remote intact
Thoughts	Slowed, reduced interests; perseverate	Often paranoid and grandiose. Bizarre ideas and topics may be expressed	Usually slowed. Preoccupied by sad and hopeless thoughts
Perception	Often normal. Hallucinations often present (frequently visual)	Visual and auditory hallucinations common	Mood congruent. Auditory hallucination in some people

ACTIVITY

Mrs M is 79 years of age and lives alone. She has hypertension, angina and a history of alcohol abuse, but recently has only needed a repeat prescription for her medication (GTN spray, atenolol and temazepam).

There is no previous psychiatric history. Her daughter, who lives nearby, contacts you to say that her mother has become confused, paranoid and aggressive. Mrs M has been shouting abuse at her neighbour, threatening him, and accusing him of trying to gas her. She has been seen wandering outside at night in a state of undress and appears to have turned night into day, often being asleep when her daughter visits.

The daughter reports that her mother's self-care is deteriorating, and that Mrs M is muddled, irritable and appears to be 'seeing things'.

Consider the following scenario:

- When you see Mrs M she seems disorientated in time and place, talking about events of many years ago. She appears paranoid, with rambling speech and fragmented thinking.
- There is poor concentration and fluctuating levels of consciousness.
- These problems apparently started about a week ago.
- On talking with Mrs M you ascertain that she decided to stop drinking about 2 weeks ago.
- Feeling tired and irritable and unable to sleep, she had increased her dose of temazepam and so ran out of these tablets about a week later.

Which of the three disorders discussed in the text is Mrs M most likely suffering from?

Depression

The elderly person who is depressed is at increased risk of developing dementia (comorbidity is estimated at 15–20%), but it is not yet clear whether depression increases vulnerability to Alzheimer's disease or is an early manifestation of the disorder. Environmental factors need careful assessment, because depression in an older person can often arise from difficulties in adapting to new surroundings or changed circumstances (e.g. bereavement or other sudden loss). Depression is also more common in chronic disease. Patients with diabetes, for example, are at greater risk of developing depression than the general population.[8]

Symptoms common to depression and dementia are listed in Box 10.2, and symptoms that differ between the two conditions are listed in Box 10.3.[9, 10]

There are other factors that might indicate a disorder other than dementia. An abrupt onset of confusion might signal a stroke or trauma. Many of these patients have a history of hypertension and other vascular risk factors. Fluctuating symptoms suggest toxins or recurrent strokes, while a gradual onset is typical of tumours.

Insidious and progressive symptoms can indicate Alzheimer's or other degenerative brain diseases. Changed gait and movement, or slowed or involuntary movements and a history of falls, may also provide important clues to the nature of the problem. Parkinsonian syndromes, normal pressure hydrocephalus, Huntington's disease, acute or chronic alcohol or drug abuse, and most strokes and mass lesions in the brain are accompanied by changes in motor behaviour in addition to possible dementia.[7]

BOX 10.3   Symptoms that differ in depression and dementia[10]
Depression
• No long history of memory loss and disorientation
• Often irritable
• Usually orientated in terms of time, place and person
• May refuse to answer questions
Dementia
• May answer questions in ways that are difficult to understand
• May have difficulty with communication, e.g. finding the right words
• Will usually have problems with orientation
• Likely to have difficulty remembering recent events
• May have problems retaining numerical information
• May be variation in level of intellectual function
• May have difficulty thinking in abstract terms

BOX 10.2   Symptoms common to depression and dementia[9]
• Cognitive problems
• Loss of energy
• Social withdrawal
• Self-neglect
• Altered sleep or appetite pattern
• Slowness of movement
• Agitation

CONCLUSION

Dementia is a particularly cruel condition, which strikes at the very core of the self and close relationships. It robs the sufferer not only of their intellectual functioning, but also of their ability to relate to those people closest to them. Diagnosing dementia early allows appropriate treatment, management and support to be given that can help delay the deterioration that results from the brain degeneration. These aspects are discussed in Chapter 11.

EVALUATION ACTIVITY

Evaluate how your knowledge of the similarities and differences between depression and dementia has changed since reading this chapter.

Reflect on what changes you will now make to your practice in view of this.

LEARNING POINTS

- Training in dementia recognition should not be confined to mental health staff
- NICE believe that as many as 700,000 people have dementia
- Several differential diagnoses exist for dementia, most notably depression and acute confusional state
- Dementia affects all groups in society equally

REFERENCES

1. Department of Health. National Service Framework for Older People. London: The Stationery Office, 2001.
2. Audit Commission. Forget Me Not: Mental Health Services for Older People. London: Audit Commission, 2000.
3. Audit Commission. Forget Me Not 2002: Developing Mental Health Services for Older People in England. London: Audit Commission, 2002.
4. Manthorpe J, Iliffe S, Eden A. Early recognition of dementia by nurses. J Adv Nurs 2003; 44(2): 183–191.
5. National Institute for Health and Clinical Excellence. http://www.nice.org.uk
6. Cayton H, Graham N, Warner J. Dementia: Alzheimer's and Other Dementias, 2nd edn. London: Class Publishing, 2002. Available at: http://www.rcpsych.ac.uk
7. Dementia Tutorial: Diagnosis and Management in Primary Care. A Primary Care Based Education/ Research Project. Available at: http://www.ucl.ac.uk/pcps/research/aps/pcop/education/workbook_nommse.pdf
8. Department of Health. National Service Framework for Diabetes. London: The Stationery Office, 2001.
9. Logie SA, et al. The diagnosis of depression in patients with dementia: use of the Cambridge Mental Disorders of the Elderly Examination (CAMDEX). Int J Geriatr Psych 1992; 7: 511–515.
10. Yesavage J. Depression in the elderly: how to recognize masked symptoms and choose appropriate therapy. Postgrad Med 1992; 91(1): 255–261.

FURTHER INFORMATION

Adams T, Manthorpe J. Dementia Care. London: Hodder & Stoughton, 2003.

Age Concern England: http://www.ageconcern.org.uk

Alzheimer's Society: http://www.alzheimers.org.uk

Carers UK: http://www.carersonline.org.uk

CJD Support Network: http://www.cjdsupport.net

Depression Alliance: http://www.depressionalliance.org.uk

Huntington's Disease Association: http://www.hda.org.uk

Kitwood T. Dementia Reconsidered: The Person Comes First. Buckingham: Open University Press, 1997.

MIND: http://www.mind.org.uk

Royal College of Psychiatrists: http://www.rcpsych.ac.uk

Chapter 11

MENTAL HEALTH
Assessment and management of dementia

Alyson Buck

LEARNING OBJECTIVES

After reading this chapter you will be able to:

- discuss assessment strategies for someone with suspected dementia
- outline medical and social care approaches to the treatment of people with dementia
- demonstrate an understanding of the role of the practice nurse in the care of people with dementia

Dementia is more than simply a matter of brain decay (see Chapter 10). Receiving a diagnosis of dementia is a devastating experience, because it strikes at the core of the person. Close relationships and the balance of roles in previously equal partnerships will shift, as one partner becomes the caregiver and the other the cared for. It is vital, therefore, that before a diagnosis is given a thorough, comprehensive assessment is completed.

ASSESSMENT IN SUSPECTED DEMENTIA

Assessment should begin with a thorough patient history and physical examination to exclude acute confusional state. Mental state examination and cognitive testing are also needed and usually precede imaging investigations such as computed tomography (CT) or magnetic resonance imaging (MRI). An electroencephalogram (EEG) is an important additional investigation that may also be used. Box 11.1 summarises the investigations that may be carried out when dementia is suspected.[1]

SCREENING TESTS

Screening tests are essential to assess cognitive function because a person with dementia can conduct a long conversation without their condition becoming apparent.

- *Mini Mental State Examination*: this is used widely and is easily administered with minimal training. It takes about 10 minutes to carry out.[2]

BOX 11.1   Investigations for suspected cases of dementia[1]

History
- Present illness, family history

Mental state examination
- Psychiatric symptoms, behavioural and personality changes

Cognitive function
- For example, Mini Mental State Examination (MMSE)[2]

Physical examination
- Blood tests including full blood count (FBC), erythrocyte sedimentation ratio (ESR), urea and electrolytes (U&E), liver function tests (LFTs), glucose, syphilis serology, thyroid function tests, vitamin B_{12} and folate, calcium, human immunodeficiency virus (HIV)
- Electrocardiogram (ECG), electroencephalogram (EEG)

Other
- Further investigations might include lumbar puncture, MRI, CT or other scans

---

- *Cognitive Impairment Test*: the six-item Cognitive Impairment Test (6CIT) is quicker to use than the MMSE and studies indicate that it may be better for identifying cases of milder dementia.[3, 4]
- *Clifton Assessment Procedure for the Elderly (CAPE)*: this usefully combines functional ability and cognitive function. Use it to profile your patient, rather than to work out their score.[5]
- *Clock-Drawing Test*: this is useful when language is a barrier to cognitive testing, but should be used with caution in a person of low educational achievement.[6]
- *Symptoms of Dementia Screener (SDS)*: this is an 11-item questionnaire designed for use by lay persons and can even be administered over the telephone.[4, 7] It can be administered by the family of a person suspected of having dementia.

None of the above tests is diagnostic but, combined with further investigations, they are the best strategy for diagnosing dementia and its various subtypes.

ACTIVITY

Gather a variety of screening tools for use with dementia and familiarise yourself with the contents.

Select one that you feel you would be able to use comfortably in everyday practice. Some screening tools can be found at: http://www.ucl.ac.uk/pcps/research/aps/pcop/education/workbook_nommse.pdf

---

MANAGEMENT OF DEMENTIA

Tom Kitwood's seminal work on care for people with dementia has changed the perception of their needs. Many people believe that a diagnosis of 'dementia' implies that nothing can be done, but in *Dementia Reconsidered* Kitwood pointed out that there is an 'old' and a 'new' culture of dementia care.[8] Better understanding of adjusting and coping strategies can help the functioning of the person with dementia. This can improve their life and that of their carers.[9, 10]

Two main theoretical approaches to dementia care have developed over recent years:[9]

- *Person-centred approach*: the 'person-centred' or 'person with dementia' approach has the patient as the primary focus. The underlying idea is that dementia occurs 'within a psychological and social frame of reference' and that recognising and maintaining this framework is an important facet of care.[11]
- *Care for the carer approach*: this approach has evolved because the 'person-centred' approach tends to lessen the significance of those who act as carers for the person with dementia. This approach has been incorporated in a variety of Government documents.[12, 13] However the exclusion of the person with dementia, through collusion between carers and practitioners, is common.

A more inclusive approach is emerging that seeks to include the affected individual and their carers in decision-making. By exploring the relationships between patient, carer and practitioner, the alliances and collusions that can impede practice can be avoided.[11]

Management of a person with dementia can be complex. A useful guide is the Initial Management of Dementia summarised as the simple four-point checklist 'DIPS' (Box 11.2).[9] Careful assessment together with appropriate treatment of any underlying illness will address the first two DIPS criteria.

BOX 11.2   Initial management of dementia: 'DIPS'

- **D**ementia: treat the cause where possible
- **I**llness: treat concurrent illness
- **P**roblem list: tackle each major problem
- **S**upport the supporters: care for the carers

ACTIVITY

Read Trevor Adams' article 'Developing an inclusive approach to dementia care'.[11]

When you are next in consultation with a person with dementia and their carer, observe the relationships occurring and see if an inclusive approach is being used.

A carer is usually prompted to come to the practice seeking help and advice by some of the wide range of problems and behavioural changes that can arise with dementia. Problems commonly experienced include:

- wandering
- agitation
- paranoia
- sleeplessness
- poor personal hygiene
- incontinence
- eating/nutritional problems
- difficulty dressing
- hallucinations
- sexually inappropriate behaviour.

Managing such problems is often very difficult, requiring a 'trial and error' approach and perseverance. Supporting and reassuring the individual and their carer is one of the most vital aspects of your work.

The following guidelines may provide reassurance:[14]

We cannot change the person. They have a brain disorder that shapes who they have become. They are not doing these things to upset or annoy you. When you try to control or change the behaviour you will most likely be unsuccessful or meet with resistance. Try to accommodate the behaviour, not control it, and remember that we can change our behaviour or the physical environment.

Behavioural problems may have an underlying physical reason – pain, adverse effects of medication, etc. Check with the doctor whether there is any treatment that might be needed.

ACTIVITY

Look at the information leaflets available for the public in your workplace.

Is there appropriate information for those with dementia and their carers, including how to access local services and support groups?

If not, obtain a selection of materials from the resources listed at the end of this chapter.

Behaviour has a purpose. Always consider what need the person might be trying to meet with their behaviour. If possible try to accommodate this.

Behaviour is triggered. The root to changing behaviour is disrupting the patterns that we create. Try a different approach or a different consequence.

What works today may not work tomorrow. Be creative and flexible in your strategies for dealing with a given issue.

Get support from others. You are not alone; there are many others with similar problems. A variety of statutory and voluntary agencies is available to help. Support groups are an invaluable source of support and the community mental health nurses (CMHNs) or local Alzheimer's society can give information on these. The Alzheimer's Society provides a range of informative material on how to deal with difficult behaviour; this can be accessed via their website or ordered in hard copy.

COMMUNICATING WITH A PERSON WITH DEMENTIA

Improving communication skills may make interaction with the person with dementia more beneficial for all concerned. These skills can be easily learned and will enhance the ability to deal with some of the difficult behaviour you may encounter (Box 11.3).

DRUG THERAPY

There is no cure for dementia but drugs can provide some relief.

Tranquillisers, antidepressants and anxiolytic drugs can relieve symptoms such as irritability, anxiety, restlessness and depression, but have side-effects.[15]

Drugs known as anticholinesterase inhibitors work by maintaining levels of acetylcholine, which affects nerve-cell communication and memory. Although these may also have side-effects, they can help improve cognitive functioning in mild to moderate dementia. They include Aricept (donepezil hydrochloride), Exelon (rivastigmine) and Reminyl (galantamine).

In moderate to severe Alzheimer's disease Ebixa (memantine hydrochloride) may protect cells from calcium damage and temporarily slow symptoms – or even the disease itself.

A specialist experienced in the management of dementia care should prescribe these drugs.[15]

Advice (2004) from the Committee for the Safety of Medicines (CSM) is that the antipsychotic drugs risperidone and olanzapine should not be used for this patient group because of an increased risk of stroke.[16]

OTHER MEASURES

Much can be done for the psychological health of people with dementia without relying on drugs, by making them feel safe and cared for and by keeping distress to a minimum (Box 11.4).

Good nutrition is essential, and vitamin supplements (particularly vitamins C, B_{12} and E) may be important.

Complementary remedies said to be helpful in dealing with Alzheimer's disease are acupuncture, aromatherapy, art, drama and music therapy, herbal remedies and massage.[17]

Some herbal remedies such as *Ginkgo biloba* are reputed to help improve memory, as are the omega-3 fatty acids found in fish oils.[17]

BOX 11.3   Ten tips for communicating with a person who has dementia[14]

1. Set a positive mood for interaction
Attitude and body language communicate thoughts and feelings more strongly than words. Set a positive mood by speaking in a pleasant and respectful manner. Facial expressions, tone of voice and physical touch can help convey the message and show a positive attitude

2. Get the person's attention
Limit distractions and noise, and before speaking ensure you have their attention. Address the person by name, identify yourself by name and use non-verbal cues to help keep them focused. If the person is seated, get down to their level and maintain eye contact

3. State your message clearly
Speak slowly, distinctly and in a reassuring tone. Keep the pitch low, and do not raise your voice higher or louder. If the person does not understand you the first time, rephrase your question or message using the same words. Avoid using jargon or abbreviations. Give the person time to respond

4. Ask simple, answerable questions
Ask one question at a time – those with simple yes/no answers work best. Avoid giving too many choices. Visual prompts and cues also help guide the response

5. Listen with your ears, eyes and heart
Be patient in waiting for a response. Watch non-verbal cues and body language and respond appropriately. Always strive to listen for the meaning and emotions that underlie the words the person uses

6. Break down activities into a series of steps
This makes many tasks more manageable. Encourage the person to do what they can, assist with things they cannot do, and remind them of things they forget

7. Distract and redirect
If the person becomes upset, try changing the subject or the environment. It is important to connect with the person before you redirect; for example, you might say 'I see you're upset, let's leave this and do...'

8. Respond with affection and reassurance
People with dementia often feel anxious, confused or unsure of themselves. Stay focused on the feelings they are demonstrating, and respond with verbal and physical expressions of comfort, support and reassurance

9. Remember the 'good old days'
This is often a soothing and affirming activity. The person may not recall events of 45 minutes ago but clearly remember things from their past. Therefore avoid asking questions that rely only on short-term memory

10. Maintain your sense of humour
Use humour whenever possible, but not at the person's expense. People with dementia will often retain their social skills and, like us all, enjoy a good laugh

The services of specialists such as neurologists, consultants in old-age psychiatry and CMHNs can be helpful, so ensure you know who they are and how to contact them.

Memory clinics have been around in Britain since the mid-1980s and are becoming more widespread. They have much to offer in the way of outpatient diagnostic and treatment services

---

Box 11.4   The role of the practice nurse

The practice nurse is in a powerful position to influence the care of people with dementia, and can do a lot to support them and their families, before and after diagnosis. The shock of receiving a diagnosis of dementia must not be underestimated and nurses must utilise their whole range of skills to support, inform and educate the patient and their family. This can be done in several ways – e.g. report to the GP any signs of increased confusion or disorientation, or changes in mood or behaviour, in the elderly people in your care.

- **Observe** these patients closely during interaction with them, looking for changes in mental and physical state. If necessary, assess them using a recognised screening tool
- **Assist in the exclusion of possible remedial causes** of increased confusion or behavioural disturbance (e.g. infection) in a person with dementia
- **Maintain open channels of communication** with the CMHNs for older people in your area and those from other disciplines involved in the person's care
- **Keep in close contact with carers,** to gain a full picture of the person's healthcare needs and social circumstances. In this way you can contribute to decision-making
- **Act as an information source** for people with dementia and their carers, and help them plan for issues or difficulties that may develop
- **Act as a referral link** to both statutory and voluntary services and organisations, especially for people with dementia who have no carer
- **Provide as much support and practical assistance to carers as possible,** and ensure they are referred to specialist agencies to help them cope with changes in their relative's functional capacity or behaviour

---

for those experiencing memory difficulties. They also have an important role in the education and training of health professionals in all aspects of dementia care. Most clinics take place in a hospital setting but some are now held in practice surgeries or in the community.

ACTIVITY

Read up on memory clinics to gain a better understanding of them.

The book edited by Curran and Wattis[4] is a useful place to start. Enquire of your local mental health services if any memory clinics operate in your area and explore the referral system for them.

CONCLUSION

The number of people with dementia is increasing and care for them must improve. There is still a tendency to see people with dementia, particularly advanced dementia, as 'non-persons'. However, even those who are severely affected can, with attention and confidence in the listener, communicate with great clarity and insight.

Small things can make a huge difference to the well-being of the individual, and towards providing the carer with the support they need. Building positive values into the care we give acknowledges that the person hidden by the fog of dementia is still there and can appreciate their surroundings.

It is possible to slow down the rate of degeneration, and help the person to be themselves for longer. Important factors are detecting dementia early, ensuring that specialist care and intervention are available, and including the cared-for and carer in decision-making.

<table>
<tr><td>

EVALUATION ACTIVITY

Reflect critically on how your attitudes towards and understanding of dementia may be affecting how you communicate with affected individuals.

Evaluate how effective any changes have been that you have made in your approach to the carers of a person with dementia.

</td><td>

LEARNING POINTS

- Screening tests are essential to assess cognitive function
- A new culture of dementia care is developing
- Managing 'behavioural problems' requires a trial and error approach
- Improved communication skills can make interaction with a person with dementia more beneficial for all concerned

</td></tr>
</table>

REFERENCES

1. Burns A, Forstl H. Alzheimer's disease. In: Butler R, Pitt B (eds), Seminars in Old-Age Psychiatry. London: Gaskell, 1998.
2. Folstein M, Folstein S, McHugh P. Mini Mental State: a practical method for grading the cognitive state of patients for the clinician. J Psychiatr Res 1975; 12: 189–198.
3. Brooke P, Bullock R. Validation of a 6-item cognitive impairment test with a view to primary care usage. Int J Geriatr Psychiatry 1999; 14: 936–940.
4. Curran S, Wattis JP (eds). Practical Management of Dementia: A Multi-professional Approach. Oxford: Radcliffe Medical, 2004.
5. Pattie A, Gilleard C. Clifton Assessment Procedure for the Elderly. Sevenoaks: Hodder & Stoughton, 1979.
6. Shulman KI. Clock drawing: is it the ideal cognitive screening test? Int J Geriatr Psychiatry 2000; 15: 548–561.
7. Mundt JC, Freed DM, Greist JH. Lay person-based screening for early detection of Alzheimer's disease: development and validation of an instrument. J Gerontol: Psychol Sci 2000; 55: 163–170.
8. Kitwood T. Dementia Reconsidered: The Person Comes First. Buckingham: Open University Press, 1997.
9. Burns A, Hope T. Clinical aspects of the dementias of old age. In: Butler R, Pitt B (eds), Seminars in Old-Age Psychiatry. London: Gaskell, 1998.
10. Hope T, Pitt B. Management of dementia. In: Butler R, Pitt B (eds), Seminars in Old-Age Psychiatry. London: Gaskell, 1998.
11. Adams T. Developing an inclusive approach to dementia care. Practice 2003; 15: 45–53.
12. Nolan M, Davies S, Grant G. Working with Older People and their Families. Buckingham: Open University Press, 2001.
13. Department of Health. Carers National Strategy. London: The Stationery Office, 1999.
14. Family Caregiver Alliance. Caregiver's guide to understanding dementia behaviours. Available at: http://www.Caregiver.org
15. British Medical Association & Royal Pharmaceutical Society of Great Britain. British National Formulary. London: BMA/RPSGB, March 2004.
16. Department of Health. New advice issued on Risperidone and Olanzapine, 2004. Available at: http://www.dh.gov.uk/PublicationsAndStatistics/PressReleases/PressReleasesNotices/fs/en?CONTENT_ID=4075751&chk=f0tw6s
17. Cayton H, Graham N, Warner J. Dementia: Alzheimer's and Other Dementias, 2nd edn. London: Class Publishing, 2002. Available at: http://www.rcpsych.ac.uk

FURTHER INFORMATION

Adams T, Manthorpe J. Dementia Care. London: Hodder & Stoughton, 2003.

Websites

Age Concern England: http://www.ageconcern.org.uk

Alzheimer's Society: http://www.alzheimers.org.uk

Carers UK: http://www.carersonline.org.uk

CJD Support Network: http://www.cjdsupport.net

Depression Alliance: http://www.depressionalliance.org.uk

Huntington's Disease Association: http://www.hda.org.uk

MIND: http://www.mind.org.uk

Royal College of Psychiatrists: http://www.rcpsych.ac.uk

Chapter 12

MENTAL HEALTH
Suicide and self-harm

Alyson Buck

LEARNING OBJECTIVES

After reading this chapter you will be able to:

- define the terms 'suicide' and 'self-harm'
- outline the epidemiology of suicide and self-harm
- understand why people might harm themselves
- discuss current strategies for reducing suicide and self-harming behaviour
- outline what to do when faced with an individual who is expressing suicidal/ self-harming ideas

It is a troubling moment in a nurse's career when a patient confides that they want to end their life, or that the injuries for which they are being treated have been self-inflicted. Reactions can encompass shock, horror, disbelief, disgust, fear or sympathy and empathy. However, if a person has summoned up the courage and energy to tell us about his or her suicidal thoughts or self-harming behaviour, we need to listen fully and openly so that we can provide the best care possible.

Many people who indulge in self-harming behaviour or make attempts on their life endure less than ideal treatment from the so-called 'caring services'.[1,2] It is important to remember that people who harm themselves are in deep distress, and their behaviour is actually often part of an effort to stay alive. It would be unrealistic to expect all practice nurses to possess the necessary skills and knowledge to assess and work with patients who self-harm on an ongoing basis. Nevertheless, you must be sufficiently aware to detect where there may be a problem, and to refer individuals on to appropriate specialist services.

EPIDEMIOLOGY OF SUICIDE

Suicide has been defined as 'a fatal act of deliberate self-harm undertaken with more or less conscious self-destructive intent, however vague and ambiguous'.[3] It is the leading cause of death in men aged 15–24 years, and the second most common cause of death among people aged under 35 years.[4] In 2004, 5,554 people committed suicide in the UK; this equates to 15 people a day, or one person every 96 minutes. Of these, 4,086 were male and 1,468 female.[5]

Reduction of the suicide rate is therefore a major public health issue, and a longstanding priority in mental health care. The White Paper *Saving Lives: Our Healthier Nation* set a target for 2010 of reducing the death rate from suicide and undetermined injury by at least one-fifth.[6] Subsequent documents have outlined strategies to improve practice.[4, 7]

The two most common methods by which people end their lives are by hanging themselves and by taking an overdose.

Overdose

The main drugs used in overdose are antidepressants, paracetamol and aspirin compounds, and coproxamol, often taken with alcohol. Restricting the availability of these drugs over the counter has led to some reduction in their use for suicide.[8]

Carbon monoxide poisoning

The proportion of suicides by carbon monoxide (CO) poisoning (inhaling car exhaust fumes) has decreased over the past 10 years – probably as a result of the increased use in vehicle exhaust systems of catalytic converters, which have reduced CO emissions.

Risk factors

Some risk factors positively related to suicide are listed in Box 12.1.

SELF-HARM

Self-harm (an act of self-injury) can take many forms, from an overdose of medication or self-poisoning to scratching, cutting and inserting objects into the body or wounds.

Self-harm is one of the top five reasons for acute medical admissions for men and women, and may account for more than 170,000 hospital attendances each year.[9] Statistics can be misleading, because people are often unwilling to admit to injuring themselves, but the numbers do seem to be rising.

ACTIVITY

Consider the statements below. Do you believe them to be true?

- People who talk about committing suicide do not go on to do so
- People who deliberately harm themselves are seeking attention
- Everyone who harms themselves is depressed
- People who really want to kill themselves will do so whatever you try to do to help
- Once people start to harm themselves, they are beyond help
- Asking someone if they feel like killing themself will put the idea into their head
- People who deliberately harm themselves will not commit suicide

---

BOX 12.1   Risk factors associated with suicide[10]

- **Age**: incidence increases with age. In recent years, the incidence in adult men up to 45 years of age has been increasing
- **Gender**: the rate is around three times higher in men than women at all ages
- **Race**: incidence is higher among the white population, but young Asian women are also at increased risk
- **Marital/employment status**: more common among divorced, single or widowed individuals, those living alone or homeless, and the unemployed
- **Occupation**: risk is higher for those in certain professions (e.g. farming, dentistry, medicine), possibly because of ready access to more lethal methods
- **Loss/bereavement**: incidence is higher among those who have suffered a recent loss, e.g. of job, partner or health (such as recent diagnosis of chronic or terminal illness such as HIV or cancer)
- **Seasonal variation**: incidence is generally higher in spring (among prisoners it is higher in autumn)
- **Deliberate self-harm**: a previous or current history of self-harm increases the risk
- **Mental illness**: incidence is higher in patients who have a current episode of mental illness or have recently been discharged from inpatient care
- **Social support**: those with poor social support are at greater risk
- **Substance misuse, forensic history**: a history of substance misuse or violent crime increases risk
- **Biological factors**: a family history of suicide increases the risk

---

It is a problem that affects more women than men (except in the prison population) and tends to involve more young people. A significant number of people who self-harm come from minority groups, who may be discriminated against within society. Those with a mental illness are at increased risk of self-harm.

ASSOCIATION BETWEEN SELF-HARM AND SUICIDE

Self-harm also has a strong association with suicide (Box 12.2). About one-quarter of all people who commit suicide have attended hospital following an act of self-harm in the preceding 12 months, and people who regularly self-harm as a way of coping are at increased risk of suicide. Substantial numbers of elderly people self-harm, and these individuals have a high level of suicidal intent.[10, 11]

BOX 12.2   A guide to terminology

- The terms *self-harm*, *deliberate self-harm*, *parasuicide* and *attempted suicide* are often used interchangeably, but do not describe the same actions. The main distinguishing factor is intent
- If, at the time of self-harming behaviour, *a person intends to take their own life but is thwarted* in that attempt (by a problem with the method or by being interrupted or treated in time), then the incident is an *attempted (but failed) suicide*
- If *the harm is inflicted* for any other reason, then it is *self-injurious (or self-harming) behaviour*, and is likely to be repeated

---

WHY DO PEOPLE SELF-HARM?

Self-harming behaviour is difficult to understand and explain. Not all people who attend with self-inflicted injuries want to kill themselves – many more people self-harm than commit suicide.

Most people do not hurt themselves so badly as to risk their lives. Their actions are a way of dealing with unbearable feelings. These may be painful emotions that, without an outlet, get directed inwards, and self-injury can be a way for individuals to express their pain and anger and to punish themselves.

A person who is self-harming may be using the only way they know to communicate their feelings to others and to try to get the care and comfort they need. However upsetting their behaviour may be, they are not necessarily intending to upset others.

Self-injury may also be a person's way of attempting to get some control over their life. Many people who self-harm will have been abused – sexually, physically or emotionally. They may have been neglected or separated from someone they loved, been bullied, or put into care, hospital or prison. They may not have had the support they needed to deal with the problem at the time, and might never have had the chance to tell anyone what happened to them. Their self-esteem may be low and they may be unable to talk about their emotions. For some, self-harm is a way of coping with inner voices.

Feeling helpless or powerless is an important factor in suicidal and self-harming behaviour. Young people often feel under great pressure from their family, school and peer group to conform or to excel. If they feel there is little chance of living up to these expectations, they may express their concerns through aggression and self-destructiveness.

ACTIVITY

Consider the patients in your care. How many of these demonstrate self-harming behaviour?

Select one whom you know to be a repeated self-harmer. What is your attitude towards this person, and why?

RESPONDING TO SELF-HARM

Because it is hard to understand, self-harm is often described as attention-seeking and manipulative behaviour. There are also many myths and misconceptions about it (Table 12.1), and it can provoke mistrust or fear. Health professionals often feel helpless or angry when faced with a person's self-inflicted wounds, and our own feelings may cause us to blame rather than support them.

Whether the injuries are minor or severe, self-harm must be taken seriously and appropriate help and support offered. People who self-harm are unlikely to be able to sort out their problems on their own. The National Institute for Health and Clinical Excellence (NICE) guidelines on self-harm (2004) focus on the management and secondary prevention of self-harm in primary and secondary care, stating that: 'primary care has an important role in the assessment and treatment of people who self harm ...' and should establish 'the likely physical risk and the person's emotional and mental state, in an atmosphere of respect and understanding'.[9]

It is the responsibility of each nurse to ensure that their own approach is sensitive and non-judgemental (Box 12.3). It is important for the person to be assessed by specialist services as soon as possible, so make sure that you know where your local mental health teams are and how patients access the crisis-resolution services.

Assessment will indicate ways to help a person who self-harms. Many will have a diagnosable mental illness, but many others attribute their self-harm to social factors; interventions should take motivating factors into account.

Therapy

Formal therapeutic interventions include the use of crisis cards, problem-solving therapy, dialectical behaviour therapy and brief therapy.[13–16]

Other interventions might include individual counselling, which can help people look at the

TABLE 12.1 Self harm: myths and misconceptions[12]

Myth	Experience of self-harmers
It is attention seeking	There are many easier, less painful and less degrading ways of attracting attention
It is a borderline personality disorder	Self-injury is not a diagnosis, it is a symptom of underlying distress
They are manipulative	Self-harm is mostly a private activity. Most professional carers will see only a few of the self-inflicted injuries: generally it is not about the effect on others
They are usually hysterical women under 30 and will grow out of it	The difference in rate of self-harm between men and women is decreasing. There is no evidence to show people grow out of it. It is neither a behavioural nor developmental disorder
As it is self-inflicted, it is not serious	Staff perception of how severe the wound is will not tell them how bad the person feels. Not all forms of self-harm will be seen, as individuals have many ways of expressing their distress
They either enjoy pain or they cannot feel it	Each person has their own threshold for pain. The loss of sensation some people feel when self-harming usually returns shortly after the act. By the time the person receives treatment the level of pain is often increased
Do not waste your time with them, they have been doing it for years	A long history of self-harm will often result in the person being considered a hopeless case. It is assumed the person is incurable
It is tension relieving	This is rarely the only pressure to self-harm, as each individual has their own trigger point

BOX 12.3 The role of the practice nurse

- **People who self-harm** often feel isolated and in despair. Knowing that others are there for them, despite what they are doing to themselves, can make all the difference. Practice nurses are in the front line of care, and can help self-harming individuals by their approach and willingness to engage with them
- **Try not to be afraid** – the patient is harming themself, not you
- **Make time to listen and try to understand** – this is one of the most important things you can do. There is no need to find solutions. Simply accept the person as they are, even though you find the self-harm upsetting
- **Try to avoid** criticising the person, attempting to control their behaviour or showing how anxious you are, however hard this may seem. They are unlikely to be able to stop self-harming immediately, and your actions may drive them to self-harm in secret
- **Do not show anger or disgust** if a person shows you evidence of their self-harm. Behave in a caring way as you would with anyone who is ill or injured
- **Find out all you can** about self-harm and about sources of help, so that you can offer suggestions that are appropriate and try to support the person while they find alternative ways of coping. Encourage any positive steps they take, even if they are continuing to self-harm
- **Try to persuade the person to see the GP for help and referral** – if they are unwilling to do this, you might suggest they contact one of the helplines listed at the end of this chapter
- **Above all, try to be patient** – the urge to inflict self-harm may take months or even years to overcome

underlying reasons for their self-harm and find more appropriate ways to express their feelings. Therapy or support groups enable people to share their thoughts and feelings with others who have had similar experiences, and to support each other to find new ways of coping. Creative arts therapies often provide a good way to express feelings that are too difficult or painful to talk about.

Practical help with benefits, accommodation, training or employment can help people find a way out of a damaging situation (e.g. a relationship with an abusive partner) or get back on their feet.

A practice nurse can help by means of supportive discussions with the patient about finding alternative ways to cope with stresses that can trigger self-harm.

Crisis support is important because many people need some sort of outside support when in distress – whether a place to go where they will feel safe and cared for, or a telephone number to ring. All mental health trusts should offer crisis resolution services, drop-in centres and mental health liaison services.

CONCLUSION

Of the many people who self-harm on a regular basis, a significant number will end up killing themselves. Suicide is a devastating event that causes considerable distress, for family and carers (who will need support – see Further Information section) and for health professionals. The issue is everyone's responsibility and the implications for practice are far-reaching. By remembering that people who self-harm are often in deep mental anguish, and developing a collaborative approach to care, service providers can ensure they offer swift, effective help.

REFERENCES

1. Bywaters P, Rolfe A. Look Beyond the Scars: Understanding and Responding to Self-injury and Self-harm. Available at: http://www.nch.org.uk

2. Starr D. Understanding those who self-mutilate. J Psychosoc Nurs Ment Health Serv 2004; 42(6): 32–40.

3. Gelder M, Lopez-Ibor J, Andreason N. New Oxford Textbook of Psychiatry. Oxford: Oxford University Press, 2003.
4. Department of Health. National Service Framework for Mental Health. London: Department of Health, 1999.
5. Samaritans. Available at: http://www.samaritans.org.uk
6. Department of Health. Saving Lives: Our Healthier Nation. London: The Stationery Office, 1999.
7. National Institute for Mental Health in England. Suicide Prevention Strategy for England: Annual Report on progress 2005. London: NIMH, 2006.
8. National Electronic Library for Mental Health. Available at: http://www.library.nhs.uk/mentalhealth
9. National Collaborating Centre for Mental Health. Self-harm: The Short-term Physical and Psychological Management and Secondary Prevention of Self-harm in Primary and Secondary Care. NICE Clinical Guideline No. 16. London: National Institute for Health and Clinical Excellence, 2004. Available at: http://www.nice.org.uk
10. Department of Health. Five-year Report of the National Confidential Inquiry into Suicide and Homicide by People with Mental Illness. London: The Stationery Office, 2001.
11. Royal College of Psychiatrists. Deliberate Self Harm among Elderly indicates High Suicide Intent [press release]. London: RCP, 2004. Available at: http://www.rcpsych.ac.uk
12. Self-harm: Myths and Common Sense. Available at: http://www.selfharmuk.org/index.asp
13. Morgan HG, Jones EM, Owen JH. Secondary prevention of non-fatal deliberate self-harm. The green card study. Br J Psychiatry 1993; 163: 111–112.
14. NHS Centre for Reviews and Dissemination. Deliberate self-harm. Effective Health Care 1998; 4(6): 1–12.
15. Lineham M. Cognitive Behavioural Treatment of Borderline Personality Disorder. New York: Guildford Press, 1993.
16. De Shazer S. Keys to Solution in Brief Therapy. New York: Norton, 1985.

FURTHER INFORMATION

Bristol Crisis Service for Women: telephone support for any woman in distress anywhere in the UK. National Helpline 0117 925 1119 (Friday and Saturday 9 p.m. to 12.30 a.m., Sunday 6–9 p.m.); http://www.users.zetnet.co.uk/BCSW

Cruse Bereavement Care: many branches have volunteers trained to help people bereaved by suicide and bereaved children. National bereavement helpline 0870 167 1677 and local branches. http://www.crusebereavementcare.org.uk

National Self-Harm Network: campaigns for a better understanding of self-harm and provides a free information pack. http://www.nshn.co.uk

Samaritans: 24-hour helpline 08457 90 90 90; http://www.samaritans.org.uk

SANE: a national mental health helpline providing information and support for people with mental health problems and those who support them. SANELINE 0845 767 8000 (every day, 12 p.m. to 2 a.m.); http://www.sane.org.uk

Self Harm Alliance: national survivor-led voluntary group supporting any person affected by self-harm. Helpline 01242 578820 (Tuesday and Sunday 6–7 p.m., Thursday 11 a.m. to 1 p.m.); http://www.selfharmalliance.org

Deliberate Self-harm in Young People: factsheet for parents and teachers, produced by the Royal College of Psychiatrists, which discusses what you can do to help, and lists sources of further information. http://www.rcpsych.ac.uk/mentalhealthinformation/mentalhealthandgrowingup/self-harminyoungpeople.aspx

NCH – Self-Harm: Look Beyond the Scars: frequently asked questions, information and resources about self-harm, especially for children and young people who are self-harming, or for their families and friends. http://www.nch.org.uk/selfharm

Self-Injury, Abuse & Trauma Resource Directory: lists self-injury, abuse, and trauma resources. http://www.self-injury-abuse-trauma-directory.info

Young People and Self-Harm: aims to provide information about initiatives in this area, provide resources to those who are affected by the issue of deliberate self-harm among young people, and to provide support to policy-makers and professionals. http://www.selfharm.org.uk

Chapter 13

GASTROINTESTINAL DISORDERS
Dyspepsia

Patricia Brown

CHAPTER CONTENTS

LEARNING OBJECTIVES

After reading this chapter you will be able to:

- discuss the incidence and causes of dyspepsia
- outline the main signs and symptoms of GORD and peptic ulcers
- outline and discuss the treatment and management of GORD and peptic ulcers
- identify when a patient has alarm features and requires urgent referral

Dyspepsia (indigestion) is a common complaint and may be described in many ways by patients.[1–4] Patients' symptoms may include all or some of those listed in Box 13.1.

ACTIVITY

Look in your practice waiting room to see whether leaflets on dyspepsia/heartburn are available for patients to take home with them. If they are, review the information and advice within them.

PREVALENCE AND CAUSES

According to the British Society of Gastroenterology (BSG), 21–41% of the UK population have dyspepsia.[1,2] Of these, 25% will seek help from

---

BOX 13.1   Symptoms of dyspepsia

- Heartburn
- Bloating
- Nausea
- Epigastric discomfort

---

their GP, a figure which suggests that up to 4% of GP consultations will be for dyspepsia. Dyspepsia has several possible causes (Box 13.2), and the cause must be correctly identified in the individual patient to ensure that he or she is treated and referred to specialists appropriately.

GASTRO-OESOPHAGEAL REFLUX DISEASE

Of all patients seeking medical advice, 10–17% are suffering from gastro-oesophageal reflux disease (GORD).[2] The main symptom of GORD is frequent heartburn,[1,3] which may be described as a burning feeling that radiates up towards the heart. The sensation of heartburn occurs when small amounts of acid present in the stomach (where it is necessary to digest food)[3,5] rise up into the oesophagus. Unlike the stomach, the oesophagus does not have a protective lining, hence the discomfort when this acid reflux occurs. It is recognised that permanent damage can occur if GORD is untreated or insufficiently treated.[4] Continued ulceration can develop into an irreversible condition known as Barrett's oesophagitis, which is associated with a 40-fold increase in the risk of developing oesophageal cancer.[4] There are circumstances in which reflux of acid into the oesophagus is more likely to occur (Box 13.3).[3,5]

PEPTIC ULCERS

A gastric ulcer is an erosion of the lining of the stomach, and a duodenal ulcer is an erosion of the lining of the duodenum; the term peptic ulcer includes both gastric and duodenal ulcers.[2,6-8]

Duodenal ulcers are said to affect four times as many men as women,[3] but there seems to be a trend towards equal prevalence in both sexes; this brings duodenal ulcers in line with gastric ulcers, which are more or less equally distributed between men and women.[2,3,9] Duodenal ulcers are two to three times more common than gastric ulcers, and around 10–15% of the population will develop a duodenal ulcer. Duodenal ulcers are more common in the north of England and in Scotland, and both gastric and duodenal ulcers are more common in older people.

Of patients with a peptic ulcer, 10–15% will complain of dyspepsia. Other symptoms include epigastric pain, which may be described by the patient as sharp, dull or penetrating, and may radiate into the back. Additionally, some patients may experience a feeling of hunger. Furthermore, up to 40% of patients with a peptic ulcer may complain of bloating and belching. Epigastric pain may occur 2–3 hours after meals and may wake the patient during the night. This pain may be worse when the stomach is empty and may be relieved for a short time by food, milk or antacids. A number of complications can arise as a result of peptic ulceration (Box 13.4).

BOX 13.2   Causes of dyspepsia

- Gastro-oesophageal reflux disease (GORD)
- Functional dyspepsia (non-ulcer dyspepsia)
- Peptic ulcer
- Gastric carcinoma
- Gallstones

BOX 13.3   Factors that may precipitate gastro-oesophageal reflux disease (GORD)

- Pregnancy
- Smoking
- Large meals (especially near bedtime)
- Being overweight

BOX 13.4   Complications of peptic ulcer

- Gastrointestinal bleeding (mortality ca. 5%)
- Pyloric stenosis
- Perforation
- Malignant change (gastric ulcers only)

Most duodenal ulcers (90–95%) and gastric ulcers (70%) are associated with the bacterium *Helicobacter pylori*.[1–3, 6, 9, 10] Most of the remainder are caused by non-steroidal anti-inflammatory drugs (NSAIDs), such as ibuprofen.[7, 10] Peptic ulcer is rare in the absence of *H. pylori* infection or NSAID use.

ACTIVITY

Find out the signs, symptoms and management of each of the possible complications of a peptic ulcer.

FUNCTIONAL DYSPEPSIA

Functional dyspepsia, or non-ulcer dyspepsia,[3, 6] are terms used when no cause can be found for an individual's dyspepsia. Examination by endoscopy generally finds nothing abnormal, or only irrelevant abnormalities such as gastric erythema. In about 50% of patients with functional dyspepsia, a test for the presence of *H. pylori* will be positive. Smoking and alcohol do not appear to worsen functional dyspepsia, but caffeine has been reported to aggravate the symptoms.

INVESTIGATIONS IN DYSPEPSIA

Two-thirds of patients with upper gastrointestinal symptoms will complain of heartburn and pain,[3, 6, 9, 11] and it is essential for patients who need further investigations to be distinguished from those for whom more conservative treatment is appropriate.

It is important to gather a detailed history from the patient and, in particular, to ask how often pain occurs and whether they have been able to identify any precipitating factors.

The purpose of investigations in the patient with dyspepsia is to help identify or rule out possible causes (Box 13.5).

TESTING FOR *HELICOBACTER PYLORI*

A blood test can identify *H. pylori* infection because, once the body has been exposed to the bacterium, antibodies to it will be detectable in the blood.[6, 7, 10] However, the test cannot distinguish between current and previous infection. A carbon-13 urea breath test (CUBT) will show whether or not *H. pylori* urease activity is occurring in the stomach. Additionally, assays are available that detect antigen derived from *H. pylori* in stool samples.

The National Institute for Health and Clinical Excellence (NICE) guidance on the management of dyspepsia recommends using a carbon-13 urea breath test or a stool antigen test for initial detection of *H. pylori*.[1]

ACTIVITY

Find out about breath testing for the detection of *H. pylori* and what the patient and nurse/GP have to do when a breath test is performed.

BOX 13.5   Investigations in dyspepsia

- Tests for the presence of *H. pylori*:
  - blood test
  - breath test
  - faecal antigen test
- Endoscopy when indicated (see text)
- Full blood count
- Ultrasound scan to identify gallstones

ENDOSCOPY

The need for cost-effective use of resources makes it essential to consider carefully which patients presenting with dyspepsia should be referred for endoscopy. It is important to diagnose gastric carcinoma as early as possible, because treatment is so effective, and of patients with gastric carcinoma 60–90% will complain of dyspepsia.[1, 2] However, fewer than 2% of all patients referred for endoscopy are found to have a gastric carcinoma.

Guidelines from NICE recommend urgent specialist referral for endoscopic investigation in patients of any age with dyspepsia who present with any of the alarm symptoms listed in Box 13.6, which indicate a risk of malignancy.

Routine endoscopic investigation is considered unnecessary for patients of any age with dyspepsia but without alarm signs. However, for patients over 55 years old endoscopy should be considered if symptoms persist despite appropriate treatment, and if there is a continuing need for NSAID treatment.

The BSG, however, advocates initial referral for endoscopy for patients over 55 years old who present with dyspepsia, even if they have no alarm signs.[1, 2] Nevertheless, they do acknowledge that this advice may change as the evidence base for this practice to continue is poor.[2]

ACTIVITY

Find out how to refer a patient for endoscopy and what happens to the patient during the examination, so that you can inform your patients appropriately.

TREATMENT

Gastro-oesophageal reflux disease

If a patient experiences heartburn several times a week, it is unlikely to get better without treat-

---

BOX 13.6 Alarm symptoms indicating a risk of malignancy in a patient with dyspepsia

- Evidence of chronic gastrointestinal bleeding (anaemia)
- Progressive unintentional weight loss
- Progressive dysphagia (difficulty swallowing)
- Persistent vomiting
- Unexplained iron-deficiency anaemia
- Epigastric mass
- Suspicious barium meal appearance
- Previous gastric surgery
- Previous gastric ulcer

---

ment. Drug treatment does not cure GORD, but it can help patients feel better and help the oesophagus to heal. If treatment is stopped, symptoms are likely to recur.

The NICE guidance on the management of dyspepsia states that the treatment for GORD is a full dose of a proton pump inhibitor (PPI) for 1–2 months, after which the dose is reduced to the lowest that maintains control of the patient's symptoms.[1, 2, 4, 10, 12]

PPIs reduce gastric acid secretion and the prescriber can choose between omeprazole (Losec), lansoprazole (Zoton), rabeprazole (Pariet), pantoprazole (Protium) and esomeprazole (Nexium).

H_2 receptor antagonists (H_2 blockers) also reduce gastric acid secretion, but symptom control is not achieved as quickly as with PPI therapy. H_2 blockers available are ranitidine (Zantac), nizatidine (Axid), famotidine (Pepcid) and cimetidine (Tagamet), some of which can be bought over the counter (OTC) at pharmacies.

Antacids and/or alginates available from a pharmacist seem to help some people with mild symptoms. After initial PPI therapy for GORD has been stepped down to the lowest effective dose, a return to self-treatment with antacid and/or alginate therapy (prescribed or purchased OTC and taken as required) may be appropriate.

Peptic ulcer disease

Eradication of *H. pylori* is a cornerstone of treatment for peptic ulcer disease.

Non–ulcer dyspepsia

Treatment for non-ulcer dyspepsia is generally with anti-secretory drugs (PPIs and H_2 blockers).

Uninvestigated dyspepsia

There has been recent reconsideration of the approach to treatment for patients who present for the first time with dyspepsia and have not been investigated previously. The initial strategy is now to try either full-dose PPI for 1 month or to test for and treat *H. pylori*, there being insufficient evidence to determine which option should be tried first, with the other treatment being offered if symptoms persist or return.[1, 2]

Patients with dyspepsia should be given advice as to how their dyspepsia may be reduced. Lifestyle advice centres around discussion on healthy eating, weight reduction and smoking cessation.[1, 2] They should also be advised to avoid any foods or drink known to precipitate their dyspepsia. It is imperative that patients understand their medication and why they are taking it, so that they will be more likely to take it as advised. In those patients with peptic ulcer who are *H. pylori* negative, it may be necessary to reconsider continuing their NSAID therapy.

FOLLOW–UP IN PEPTIC ULCER DISEASE

Following *H. pylori* eradication treatment, patients who are asymptomatic do not need a repeat breath test or endoscopy. In all patients where symptoms persist or recur, it is recommended that a repeat urea breath test should be performed, at least 1 month after *H. pylori* eradication treatment has been completed. If the repeat breath test is negative, no further treatment is necessary. However, where it is positive a second course of eradication therapy may be given.

Treatment with PPIs and H_2 blockers should be stopped for a minimum of 2 weeks before *H. pylori* testing or endoscopy.

CONCLUSION

Dyspepsia is a common complaint. As a practice nurse you are an integral part of the multi-disciplinary team, and as such it is important that you are aware of the causes, investigations and management of dyspepsia. Only then will you be able to ensure that your patients are offered appropriate investigations and that the necessary treatment is prescribed.

Patients should be advised how to reduce their dyspepsia. Lifestyle advice is centred around healthy eating, weight reduction and smoking cessation. Patients should avoid any foods or drinks known to precipitate their dyspepsia. Patients must understand their medication and why they are taking it, as this increases compliance. In those patients with peptic ulcer who are *H. pylori* negative, it may be necessary to reconsider continuing their NSAID therapy.

EVALUATION ACTIVITY

Reflect critically on the care of people with dyspepsia within your practice.

Indentify strengths in clinical care and areas for future development.

LEARNING POINTS

- You should be able to identify the main causes of dyspepsia
- Be aware of the alarm symptoms that indicate a risk of malignancy in a patient with dyspepsia
- Be aware of the patient's journey through the investigations for dyspepsia
- Familiarise yourself with the treatments available for GORD/peptic ulcer disease

---

REFERENCES

1. National Institute for Health and Clinical Excellence. Clinical Guideline 17. Dyspepsia: Managing Dyspepsia in Adults in Primary Care. London: NICE, 2004. Available at: http://www.nice.org.uk
2. British Society of Gastroenterology. Guidelines in Gastroenterology: Dyspepsia Management Guidelines. London: BSG, 2004. Available at: http://www.bsg.org.uk
3. Talley J. Non-ulcer dyspepsia. Am Phys 2000; May: 1407–1416.
4. Smith J. Dyspepsia. Philadelphia: Mosby, 2002.
5. Marieb E. Human Anatomy and Physiology. London: Baillière Tindall, 2003.
6. Lassen A, Hallas J, Schaffalitzky de Muckadell O. *Helicobacter pylori* test and eradicate versus prompt endoscopy for management of dyspeptic patients: 6.7 year follow-up of a randomized trial. Gut 2004; 53: 1758–1763.
7. Waller D, Renwick A, Hillier K. Medical Pharmacology and Therapeutics. Edinburgh: Saunders, 2001.
8. The REflux FORuM (REFORM). Dyspepsia: Managing Adult Patients in Primary Care. REflux FORuM (REFORM), 2004. Available at: http://www.refluxforum.co.uk
9. British Medical Association & Royal Pharmaceutical Society of Great Britain. British National Formulary (BNF) 49. London: BMA & RPSGB, September 2004.
10. Jones RH. Approaches to uninvestigated dyspepsia. Gut 2002; 50(Suppl 4): iv42–iv46.
11. Thompson W. Dyspepsia. London: Churchill Livingstone, 2001.
12. Manes G, Menchise A, de Nucci C, Balanzo A. Empirical prescribing for dyspepsia: randomized controlled trial of test and treat versus omeprazole treatment. BMJ 2003; 326: 1118.

FURTHER INFORMATION

British Society of Gastroenterology: 3 St. Andrew's Place, Regents Park, London NW1 4LB; http://www.bsg.org.uk

Gut (International Journal of Gastroenterology and Hepatology): BMJ Journals Department, BMA House, Tavistock Square, London WC1H 9JP; http://gut.bmjjournals.com

Digestive Disorders Foundation: patient information leaflets and factsheets on many digestive disorders (bulk copies available). PO Box 251, Edgware, Middlesex HA8 6HG; http://www.digestivedisorders.org.uk

REFORM (REflux FORuM): provides links to other relevant sites. http://www.refluxforum.co.uk

Chapter 14

GASTROINTESTINAL DISORDERS
Irritable bowel syndrome

Graham Harris

CHAPTER CONTENTS

LEARNING OBJECTIVES

After reading this chapter you will be able to:

- give an explanation of the condition irritable bowel syndrome (IBS)
- discuss how the condition may manifest and the kinds of problems patients may experience
- discuss the diagnosis and management of the condition and outline strategies that can help to minimise or overcome associated problems

Those who experience irritable bowel syndrome (IBS) have described it as a 'nightmare' and as 'agony'.[1,2] Although this may seem melodramatic, it is important not to underestimate the misery caused by the combination of pain, bloating and other distressing symptoms. Symptoms may range from mild to severe, and accepting how the patient describes their experiences is critical to successful treatment.[3,4]

Practice nurses are often singled out when a patient wants to discuss symptoms perceived as

ACTIVITY

Think about the term 'IBS'. What does it mean to you? What might it mean to a patient? How would you explain it to a person who is unfamiliar with the term?

embarrassing or 'impolite'. This is particularly noticeable in gastrointestinal (GI) disorders and means that an understanding of GI conditions, including IBS, is an essential part of a practice nurse's repertoire of knowledge and skills.

IBS: EXPLORING THE TERMS

IBS has been described as 'a common condition in which recurrent abdominal pain with constipation and/or diarrhoea continues for years without any general deterioration in health'.[5] As a definite prognosis is not possible, it may be less pessimistic and more helpful to say that symptoms 'may persist for some time'.

Many patients will have read about the condition. Its various names such as spastic colon, mucous colitis and functional bowel disorder all give an indication of the nature of the problem but, as IBS is by far the most common name, it is better to use this.[6]

The word 'irritable' refers to muscular reactions in the intestine that result in abnormal contractions. In turn, the contractions are responsible for the three main symptoms: abdominal pain, diarrhoea and constipation.[6–8] They are recurrent, and, as already noted, may continue for some time.

WHAT CAUSES IBS?

IBS is sometimes considered to be a condition of modern living – it is thought that stress and anxiety, possibly in combination with dietary factors and allergies, are responsible.[3, 6, 9] Some people develop IBS when others with similar lifestyles or in similar situations do not. About 10–20% of people will date the start of their symptoms to an episode of acute gastroenteritis; in the remainder of cases, the trigger factor is uncertain.[10]

What is certain, however, is that IBS occurs mostly in younger and mid-life age groups, and is more often reported by women.[3, 4, 6, 9] Recent figures suggest that in Britain about 13% of women are affected, compared with 5% of men.[10] This equates with a total of around 8 million UK sufferers.[4, 6] Of these only 25% will consult a doctor about their problems, even though for around 50% of all attendances at GI outpatient departments, IBS is likely to be the cause.[3]

An average of 17 days' work is lost per sufferer per year.[6] Given that an estimated one in five adults in industrialised countries has the condition, this equates to considerable financial deficit and human suffering.

PRESENTATION AND SYMPTOMS

Like all syndromes, IBS is characterised by a collection of symptoms with similar features that occur together in a recognisable pattern.[11] In this case, the pattern is one of alternating diarrhoea and constipation with abdominal pain, bloating and characteristic stools (Box 14.1).[3, 10] Many patients say that their pain is relieved with bowel movement and that more frequent bowel movements occur with the onset of pain.[6]

However, IBS is associated with many other symptoms and non-GI features such as disturbed

---

BOX 14.1 Characteristics of bowel actions commonly reported in IBS[3]

- Small volume
- Frequent passage
- Pencil-like or similar to rabbits' motions
- Accompanied by urgency
- Typically occur in the morning

sleep and headache.[6, 12] In fact, there is a whole range of associated problems, from dysmenorrhoea to generalised pruritus (Box 14.2).

BOX 14.2   Clinical features in IBS

GI tract symptoms
- Painful constipation
- Diarrhoea
- Painful constipation and diarrhoea occurring together and accompanied by abdominal pain
- Unpredictable, erratic bowel actions – varying on daily basis
- Abdominal distension (bloating)
- Tenesmus (the frequent desire to evacuate the bowel – often without producing any significant faecal matter)
- Dyspepsia
- Borborygmi (rumbling noises caused by the movement of gas in the intestines)
- Excessive flatus

Gynaecological symptoms
- Dysmenorrhoea (painful periods)
- Dyspareunia (painful or difficult sexual intercourse – or pain following intercourse)
- Premenstrual tension

Urinary tract symptoms
- Frequency of micturition
- Urgency
- Hesitancy
- Nocturia
- Incomplete emptying of bladder

Other symptoms
- Back pain
- Pruritus (generalised itching)
- Headache
- Halitosis and/or an unpleasant taste in the mouth
- Disturbed sleep
- Constant tiredness or fatigue
- Depression
- Anxiety

The impact of symptoms can be severe. Aside from the physical problems, many sufferers have low self-esteem and feel isolated. IBS is not life-threatening but it can still mean restrictions to social activity; some will avoid travelling, and curtail sexual intercourse and leisure pursuits.[6] Some will feel depressed and may be frightened that their symptoms are indicative of more serious disease.

FACTORS IN THE DIAGNOSIS OF IBS

The diagnosis of IBS is made principally on the basis of the pattern of reported symptoms, along with some relatively simple tests and monitoring.[10] For very anxious patients it may cause concern that there is no specific investigation to confirm IBS. However, the diagnosis is not made simply by excluding other diseases. There are two sets of criteria used to establish the diagnosis: the Manning criteria and the Rome criteria.[3, 6]

The Manning criteria focus on six key features:

- abdominal pain relieved by defaecation
- diarrhoea or looser stools with the onset of abdominal pain
- more frequent stools with the onset of abdominal pain
- abdominal distension
- passage of mucus in stools
- tenesmus – the sensation of incomplete bowel evacuation.

The Rome criteria help to strengthen the diagnosis by looking at the occurrence of further signs and symptoms, such as urinary tract or gynaecological problems (see Box 14.2).[3]

ACTIVITY

Think of a patient with IBS. What tests and investigations did they require before the diagnosis was made? For what reasons were these tests undertaken?

The need to exclude other conditions may be high on the patient's agenda. They may, for example, be aware that an alteration in bowel habit can be one of the first symptoms of bowel cancer and hence be anxious that they are thoroughly investigated.

TESTS AND INVESTIGATIONS

There is a wide range of diagnostic methods available to identify and exclude organic bowel disease. These include ultrasound, radiographic and barium imaging as well as gastroscopy and colonoscopy. However, it is not always helpful to subject patients to successive, often rather unpleasant, investigations and they should not be performed routinely.[3]

In many cases, it is sufficient to take a detailed history (examined against the Manning and Rome criteria) and carry out a physical examination that includes rectal examination and sigmoidoscopy, with follow-up over a period of weeks or months.[13] The follow-up should entail the patient returning to discuss their symptoms and progress. If the symptoms are resolving, referral to a gastroenterologist may be unnecessary.

There are of course cases that prove particularly difficult. Some patients report a pattern of symptoms characteristic of IBS but, at the same time, identify clinical features not usually associated, such as pale stools or weight loss. These need separate investigation and, because IBS can mimic other disorders, other symptoms will need to be re-examined. Keeping an open mind is essential.

MANAGEMENT ISSUES

The management of irritable bowel syndrome requires consideration of a variety of factors. The aim is to encourage self-reliance on the part of the patient, wherever possible, while at the same time trying to ensure the prompt relief of symptoms. Key areas to consider include explanation and reassurance, pain management, advice on drug therapies and diet, and ongoing monitoring and support.

Explanation and reassurance

The words 'explanation' and 'reassurance' are often used in healthcare – sometimes with little empathy or understanding. To give meaningful explanations and real reassurance involves helping a person to make sense of their situation.

Initially the health professional should listen carefully, conveying their acceptance of the patient's description of their experiences by paraphrasing and summary. Sensitive questioning should be used to clarify issues and ensure mutual understanding. Giving correct information is central to this, but reassurance is rarely achieved just by reciting a definition or providing a list of 'dos' and 'don'ts'. It is far more important to hear the patient out, allowing them opportunity to ask their own questions.

Sometimes it is necessary to help 'unjumble' the various ideas, explanations and definitions that patients may have read or heard about. Fact sheets or reference to other resources such as internet sites or books may help.

Face-to-face consultation is important for the recognition of the patient's stress, anxiety and depression. As stress seems to play a part in both symptom onset and exacerbation, helping patients to become aware of their stress levels and to find ways of coping is crucial. This has been underlined by research undertaken in Australia in 1998, which showed that, for patients with unresolved high-level chronic stress, symptoms of IBS were not likely to settle at all.[14] Major chronic stressors include relationship difficulties, bullying at work and pressurised work environments.

The detection of high stress levels and depression requires sensitive, supportive interaction and a relationship of trust. Patients may identify the issues for themselves, otherwise a well-timed, well-worded question may be all that is necessary. A simple enquiry into work or home life can be a good starting point. However, it is important to be aware that such questions can provoke responses that require more time than the average consultation period.

It is often at this point that counselling and other therapies will need to be discussed. Some find relaxation through complementary therapies. Others may require more traditional psychotherapies and counselling. Close links between psychology departments and gastroenterologists have been advocated, even with joint follow-up for some patients. Practices should have identified links with local psychotherapists and counselling services, and there should be a clear protocol for patient referrals.

It has been suggested that physical activity and exercise can help to improve digestion and reduce stress.[10] This is sound advice but must be tailored to suit the individual. It is unlikely, for example, that people will engage in group sports if they are affected by embarrassing symptoms of wind or gurgling noises within their colon. Concerns about smell and noise are often paramount for sufferers, along with the fears of incontinence, both urinary and faecal.

PAIN MANAGEMENT

The pain in IBS can occur in any part of the gut (Box 14.3) and is one of the most distressing symptoms. Its management is a priority. Treatment will of course depend on pain type and severity, and some patients will require no specific medical intervention. Remedies such as a warm towel around the abdomen or hot-water bottle against the lower back may help some, while others will choose a medication such as a simple analgesic, such as paracetamol, or one of the preparations aimed at reducing bloating, such as Deflatine. Over-the-counter medications are often sufficient, but professional advice regarding side-effects may be necessary and it is worth

---

BOX 14.3   Sites/types of pain in IBS*

Oesophagus
- Heartburn – burning pain behind sternum
- Odynophagia – painful swallowing but without hold-up of food

Stomach
- Dyspepsia
- Abdominal bloating

Small bowel
- Abdominal bloating – usually subsides overnight
- Abdominal tenderness

Large bowel
- Abdominal bloating
- Right-sided abdominal pain – either low or 'tucked-up' under ribs
- Pain under left ribs (splenic flexure syndrome) – when severe may extend into left axilla
- Proctalgia fugax – severe, short stabbing pains in the rectum

Other
- Headaches
- Back pain
- Dysmenorrhoea – painful periods
- Dyspareunia – pain during/following sexual intercourse

*Adapted Rutherford.[10]

---

referring patients to the pharmacist with specific questions.

Drugs that may be prescribed include antispasmodics such as dicycloverine when abdominal cramps are a major problem. Tricyclic antidepressants are sometimes used to relieve pain in people who have not responded to other treatments.[10] In all cases, the aim is to keep the dose of the medication as low as possible and to monitor progress regularly so that the course of treatment is as short as is practicable.

Drug therapies

There is a range of drug therapies available to help with the various symptoms of IBS aside from pain, many of which can again be purchased over-the-counter. It is important, therefore, that patients are asked about any medications they may be using and their effects.

Drugs that may be used include:

- stool-softening laxatives – where constipation is a major problem, e.g. Idrolax; osmotic and bulk-forming laxatives are preferable to stimulant ones[6]
- antidiarrhoeals – where diarrhoea is a major problem, e.g. loperamide, codeine phosphate
- cholestyramine – reported to be helpful for the small proportion of IBS sufferers who have diarrhoea secondary to impaired metabolism of bile salts within the gut
- serotonin antagonists – currently under trial in IBS
- drugs for the treatment of gas and bloating, e.g. Deflatine.

As a general rule, if the patient can manage without the drug it is far better that they do so. All medications will have side-effects, so advice should be given as appropriate to enable the patient to recognise problems associated with particular drug groups.

Dietary advice

For many years, health professionals have, as a general maxim, advocated a well-balanced diet – high in fibre. And for some patients with IBS, this may be entirely appropriate. However, some research shows that wholemeal wheat and bran products may seriously exacerbate the symptoms of IBS.[15] Similarly, other research has highlighted food intolerance as a major issue in IBS, with dairy products and grains commonly incriminated.[16]

A reasonable course is to advise patients taking a low-fibre diet to increase their intake of fibre and to adjust the amount according to response. For those suffering pain and distension, but consuming a high-fibre diet, fibre intake should be reduced and the same principle of adjusting intake according to response applied.[3, 10, 15] This self-regulating approach can be adopted for patients concerned about the intake of dairy products.

There are numerous books recommending all manner of detoxifying regimens and diets for IBS. It is up to the patient to decide whether such an approach is appropriate for them and, as long as there is no serious chance of harm, they may experiment to see if one particular diet suits them.

However, it is worth encouraging patients to follow the straightforward guidance suggested by Rutherford.[10] He points out that it is often beneficial for patients to:

- consume around 3 litres of water a day
- avoid large quantities of tea, coffee, spicy foods and foods known to produce wind
- limit alcohol intake
- eat regular small amounts rather than large meals.

Support and ongoing monitoring

In some areas, practice nurses are playing a key part in providing ongoing support and monitoring of patients with IBS. Again, the idea is to promote patient self-reliance through education and advice, and in many cases this can be achieved via referrals to self-help groups or external resources such as the IBS Network (see Further Information). These groups offer befriending services for people whose symptoms are particularly severe, but it may be that the practice nurse offers telephone contact as a way of maintaining support.

Simple advice is often very welcome. Problems like peri-anal soreness from diarrhoea can be hard to deal with, so patients are often grateful for a nurse's suggestion of a suitable application. The same applies for problems such as constipation; an awareness of its effects on the patient's life is necessary in order to advise on its avoidance and management.[17]

ACTIVITY

Consider your work base. Is there information about IBS available for patients to read and take away? Is there information about diet and other lifestyle changes that may help to improve symptoms?

Is it clear and easy to read?

Where is the information placed? Could it be better displayed?

Is there a self-help group for patients in your area?

Do you run a clinic or health promotion group for IBS sufferers?

What resources would you need to set up such a group or health promotion programme?

Some practitioners may recommend that patients keep a diary, and this may help to identify particular food intolerances or triggers to bouts of symptoms, such as stressful events.

Keeping things in perspective can be difficult when the patient feels there is no hope of cure. Nevertheless, the long-term outlook need not be bleak; sometimes symptoms disappear for a while, or at least significantly reduce. Of course, in many cases, the patient has to come to terms with the fact that their symptoms will occur periodically throughout their life. All the same, knowing that a well-informed practitioner is available to offer support and encouragement can be a source of much comfort.

CONCLUSION

IBS is a common condition that presents health professionals with many challenges. There are a number of treatment strategies, and practice nurses can make a real difference to the patient's experience of symptoms and offer realistic, practical and evidence-based advice and support.

EVALUATION ACTIVITY

Reflect critically on the care of people with IBS within your practice.

In light of your learning from this chapter, indentify strengths in clinical care and areas for future development.

REFERENCES

1. IBS Tales: Personal Experiences of Irritable Bowel Syndrome. Available at: http://www.ibstales.com
2. Discovery Health. The Agony of Irritable Bowel Syndrome. Available at: http://www.discoveryhealth.co.uk
3. Moriarty KJ. The irritable bowel syndrome. In: Jones DJ (ed.), ABC of Colorectal Diseases, 2nd edn. London: BMJ Books, 1999; chapter 6, pp 21–28.
4. Jones R, Lydeard S. Irritable bowel syndrome in the general population. BMJ 1992; 304: 87–90.
5. Martin EA (ed.). Concise Medical Dictionary, 3rd edn. Oxford: Oxford University Press, 1990.
6. Moriarty KJ. Understanding Irritable Bowel Syndrome. Poole: Family Doctor Publications, 2003.
7. Thompson W. Gut Reactions. Cambridge, MA: Perseus Press, 1989.
8. Mead M. Aids to General Practice, 2nd edn. Edinburgh: Churchill Livingstone, 1990.
9. Thompson WC, Heaton KW, Smyth CT, Smyth C. Irritable bowel syndrome in general practice: prevalence, characteristics, and referral. Gut 2000; 46: 78–82.
10. Rutherford D. Irritable bowel syndrome (IBS). Available at: http://www.netdoctor.co.uk/diseases/facts/irritablecolon.htm
11. Brooker C (ed.). Pocket Medical Dictionary, 15th edn. Edinburgh: Churchill Livingstone, 2003.
12. Bradford N. Men's Health Matters – The Complete A–Z of Male Health. London: Vermilion, 1995.
13. Heaton KW, Thompson WG. Irritable Bowel Syndrome. Oxford: Health Press, 1999.
14. Bennett EJ, Tennant CC, Plesse C, Badcock C, Kellow JE. Level of chronic life stress predicts clinical outcomes in irritable bowel syndrome. Gut 1998; 43: 256–261.
15. Francis CY, Whorwell PJ. Bran and irritable bowel syndrome: time for reappraisal. Lancet 1994; 344: 39–40.
16. Nanda R, James R, Smith H, Dudley CR, Jewell DP. Food intolerance and the irritable bowel syndrome. Gut 1989; 30: 1099–1104.
17. Richards S. Constipation – a common problem. Practice Nurse 2004; 10 September: 42–48.

FURTHER INFORMATION

Digestive Disorders Foundation: http://www.digestivedisorders.org.uk

IBS Network: offers membership to both people with the condition and interested professionals. It publishes a magazine *Gut Reaction* (as well as various factsheets) and coordinates local self-help groups, campaigns and e-mail discussion lists. It also offers members a 'Can't Wait Card', which can be shown in restaurants or shops. The IBS Network, Northern General Hospital, Sheffield S5 7AU; Tel: 0114 2611531; http://www.ibsnetwork.org.uk

IBS Research Appeal: http://www.IBSResearchUpdate.org

IBS Self-help Group: http://www.ibsgroup.org

Section 2

Sexual health

SECTION CONTENTS

Chapter 15

FEMALE SEXUAL HEALTH
Sexually transmitted infections

Sarah Kraszewski

LEARNING OBJECTIVES

After reading this chapter you will be able to:

- outline the national initiatives to improve sexual health
- discuss the delivery of sexual health services
- be aware of the safer sex messages and sexual health promotion issues to communicate to clients
- understand clients' needs and be able to direct them to appropriate sources for information, diagnosis and treatment
- understand current issues surrounding *Chlamydia*, and health promotion measures being undertaken to control spread, including the role of general practice
- understand the need for collaborative working with other agencies

Sexually transmitted infections (STIs) are a significant public health issue. Globally, the World Health Organisation (WHO) estimates that there are 340 million new cases of curable STIs a year,[1] while recent figures from the Health Protection Agency (HPA) indicate that in England, Wales and Northern Ireland the number of STIs rose by 4% between 2002 and 2003 (Table 15.1). In particular, the incidence of *Chlamydia*, now the most common STI diagnosed in genito-urinary medicine (GUM) clinics, rose by 9%.[2] The

TABLE 15.1   Changing prevalence of sexually transmitted infections in the UK[2]

Disease	New cases in 2002	New cases in 2003	Change (%)
Chlamydia	82,558	89,818	+9
Genital herpes	18,432	17,990	−2
Genital warts	69,569	70,883	+2
Gonorrhoea	25,065	24,309	−3
Syphilis	1,232	1,575	+28

HPA report highlights distinct variations across the country, which signal the impact of local outbreaks and the distribution of high-risk groups.[2]

The report's authors attribute part of the rise to increased public awareness causing more people to come forward for testing. However, they also acknowledge that key groups, such as gay men and young people, continue to indulge in risky sexual behaviour and require targeting to reduce the infection rates. STIs and human immuno-deficiency virus (HIV) cause an extensive range of illnesses and contribute to the burden of long-term ill health and disability in the UK.[2]

ACTIVITY

Download a copy of the *National Strategy for Sexual Health and HIV* and of the Implementation Action Plan.

Review your practice profile and note the different groups of patients. How many of these groups fall into the high-risk category for STIs?

What is the role of general practice and practice nurses in implementing the national sexual health strategy?

Discuss with your team how you can achieve the aims of the strategy for the high-risk groups.

NATIONAL STRATEGY

A *National Strategy for Sexual Health and HIV* was published for consultation in 2001, and followed in 2002 by the implementation plan.[3, 4] The strategy is ambitious, and a central theme is the participation of primary care in its delivery.[5]

OVERVIEW OF STIs

STIs are infections transmitted primarily through sexual contact, the main causative organisms being viruses, bacteria, fungi and protozoa (Table 15.2). Some are easy to diagnose and treat, others

less so, while some, such as herpes and HIV, are incurable.[1]

The most common presenting symptoms are urethral discharge, genital ulceration, and vaginal discharge with or without vulval irritation.[1] However, it is important to remember that STIs can be asymptomatic.

STIs are common and their potential impact on health services is vast. Complications can develop when sexual health is poor, and sequelae of STI include pelvic inflammatory disease (PID), abortions, infertility and neonatal blindness.[6] In addition, STI syndromes, in particular ulcerative or inflammatory conditions, are associated with the transmission of HIV. These infections can therefore have far-reaching social, physical and economic consequences.

TABLE 15.2 Causative agents of sexually transmitted infections	
Organism	Condition
Viruses	
Papillomavirus	Genital warts
Pox virus	Molluscum contagiosum
Human immunodeficiency virus	HIV-positive state; AIDS
Herpes simplex virus type 1 and (mainly) type 2	Genital herpes
Hepatitis viruses A, B and C	Hepatitis A, B and C
Bacteria	
Chlamydia trachomatis	Non-specific urethritis, pelvic infection, neonatal eye infection
Neisseria gonorrhoeae	Gonorrhoea
Treponema pallidum	Syphilis
Gardnerella vaginalis	Bacterial vaginitis
Protozoa	
Trichomonas vaginalis	Trichomoniasis
Parasites	
Sarcoptes scabiei	Scabies
Phthirus pubis	Pubic lice
Fungi	
Candida albicans	Candidiasis

changed attitudes – in those at risk, so that infection is avoided. Individuals who decide to become sexually intimate must be aware of the high prevalence of STIs and the risks associated with them. An important message to communicate is that sexual intimacy does not have to entail intercourse, and that pleasure can be gained from other forms of closeness.

Important behavioural changes to reduce STI transmission include:

- increased age at first intercourse
- discrimination in partner selection
- less frequent changes of partner
- monogamous relationships.

Biomedical interventions to prevent the acquisition of infection include use of vaccines and of condoms and dental dams (thin latex sheets placed over the genitals or anal area before oral sex, to help reduce the risk of infection).

Hepatitis A, B and C can all be transmitted sexually. Hepatitis A transmission can occur via the oro-anal route, placing recent contacts of an acute case at risk. Normal human immunoglobulin given within 14 days of exposure confers passive immunity, while hepatitis A vaccine given within 7 days provides active immunity. A booster dose at 6–12 months gives longer term immunity.

Safer sex messages

Health professionals have a responsibility to promote safer sex in addition to passing on to patients other health promotion messages.

PRIMARY PREVENTION OF STIs

Primary prevention of STIs is achieved through avoidance of risky sexual behaviour – as a result of increased knowledge and skills, together with

Both acute and chronic infection with hepatitis B carry a transmission risk. Giving hepatitis B immunoglobulin confers passive immunity, while for the high-risk client and infected contacts, active immunity can be bestowed through hepatitis B vaccination, according to manufactur-ers' guidelines. No vaccine is available for hepatitis C.

Prophylactic vaccination may be appropriate for high-risk groups, including gay and bisexual men, injecting drug users, commercial sex workers, prisoners and the household contacts of infected individuals. Screening, contact tracing and vaccination should be considered for individuals who fall into these groups and their contacts.[7, 8]

The use of condoms and dental dams should be promoted to prevent transmission of STIs, particularly HIV. Dental dams should not be used as an alternative to a condom.[7] Free condoms and dental dams are available, and it is essential that the practice nurse knows where to refer clients, particularly if the practice does not carry supplies. Remember that high-risk groups include the gay community and young people.[1]

ACTIVITY

What sexual health services are available for young people in your locality?

Where can your clients obtain free condoms (male and female) and dental dams?

How can they access this information? How is it advertised?

Consider how you display in the surgery information relating to sexual health and safer sex.

Discuss with your practice team how the practice approaches sexual health promotion. What strategies can you use as a team to improve the sexual health of your clients?

---

and *Candida albicans*. Other tests for herpes viruses and HIV will be offered according to individual need, following counselling.

Contact tracing is an important part of STI control; sexual contacts of affected individuals may be unaware of their increased risk of infection.

SECONDARY PREVENTION OF STIs

One means of secondary prevention of STIs is reducing the prevalence of bacterial STIs, through screening and treatment with antibiotics.[9] The current initiative on controlling chlamydial infection reflects this approach.

GUM clinics

GUM clinics are an established feature in the management of STIs, offering open access and confidential testing and treatment for symptomatic and asymptomatic individuals. The management provided is determined by local guidelines.

A basic screen is likely to look for *Treponema pallidum*, *Neisseria gonorrhoeae*, *Chlamydia trachomatis*, *Trichomonas vaginalis*, *Gardnerella vaginalis*

ACTIVITY

Visit the following internet sites, which provide information on safer sex. Review the sites and decide which groups they are aimed at:

- http://www.bbc.co.uk/wales/comeclean
- http://www.likeitis.org
- http://www.nhsgrampian.org/nhsgrampian/ gra_display_simple_index.jsp?pContentID=3171 &tp_applic=CCC&tp_service=Content.show&

Design an information sheet with the resource addresses to give to clients.

Undertake the quiz at http://www. teencarecenter.org/index.php?s=vital&tp=quiz

Assess its suitability for teaching your younger clients about safer sex.

ACTIVITY

Reflect on the provision of sexual services and the role of general practice, with particular reference to the issues of screening and contact tracing.

What are the implications of screening for *C. trachomatis* in general practice, without facilities to screen for other STIs that may also be present?

Find out the location and times of local GUM services. Obtain cards for patients to pick up. Consider appropriate places to leave the cards in the surgery.

How can general practice work with GUM to provide effective sexual health promotion? You may wish to visit the GUM clinic to discuss collaborative working.

Taking a sexual health history

Taking a good sexual health history requires sensitive communication skills. Trust needs to be established, and the health professional must acknowledge that people may find it difficult to discuss their sex lives. A general sexual health history will include:

- duration of any symptoms
- date of last intercourse

ACTIVITY

Reflect upon your skills in taking a sexual health history.

How do you approach this sensitive topic with your clients?

Consider specific issues that require exploration for males and females. (There is useful information in Adler et al.[1])

Study guidelines for the treatment of STIs, available at: http://www.bashh.org and http://www.who.int/docstore/hiv/STIManagemntguidelines

---

- age and sex of partner and whether casual or long-term
- use of barrier methods
- sites of exposure
- last partner change
- partner symptoms
- any history of STIs.[10]

There may be more specific issues relating to males and females.

CHLAMYDIAL INFECTION

Chlamydial infection (Box 15.1) is the most common STI in the UK. Higher rates of diagnosis are seen in young people, the infection being most

---

BOX 15.1   Signs and symptoms of chlamydial infection[5, 11]

Women
- About 80% will be asymptomatic
- Postcoital bleeding
- Intermenstrual bleeding
- Lower abdominal pain
- Dyspareunia
- Dysuria
- Purulent vaginal discharge
- Mucopurulent cervicitis and/or contact bleeding

Men
- About 50% will be asymptomatic
- Urethral discharge
- Dysuria (may be variable and so mild the patient does not notice)

Rectal infections
- Usually asymptomatic; may cause anal discharge and discomfort

Pharyngeal
- Usually asymptomatic, but may report a sore throat

common in men and women aged 16–24 years.[11] Unfortunately, few of those at risk of this infection understand what it is, even if they have heard about it.

Chlamydia is principally transmitted through vaginal intercourse, but can also be spread via oral and anal routes.[5] Sites of infection include the urethra, rectum, pharynx, conjunctiva and cervical canal; in women infection may spread upward and cause pelvic infection, and *Chlamydia* is the most common preventable cause of female infertility. Vertical transmission to neonates can occur from women with cervical infection during delivery, usually causing eye infection.

Chlamydial infection is often asymptomatic in men and women unless it leads to complications (Box 15.2), by which time treatment may be too late to stop permanent damage. A large proportion of cases remains undiagnosed, and infection may not be confined to the groups generally considered to be at risk of STIs. Asymptomatic individuals can transmit the infection.[11]

BOX 15.2   Complications of untreated chlamydial infection

In women
- Pelvic inflammatory disease
- Chronic pelvic pain
- Ectopic pregnancy (fallopian tubes damaged)
- Infertility (fallopian tubes damaged or blocked)
- Fitz–Hugh–Curtis syndrome (infectious perihepatitis)

In neonates of infected women
- Conjunctivitis and pneumonia

In men
- Epididymo-orchitis (marked pain, swelling and redness in the scrotum on one or both sides)
- Reiter's syndrome (reactive arthritis)

General
- Adult conjunctivitis
- Facilitates transmission of HIV

Testing for *Chlamydia*

Until recently testing for *Chlamydia* in women required a swab to be taken from the cervix. Now it is much easier, because new laboratory tests have been developed that can be carried out on a urine sample or on a swab that the woman can insert into the vagina herself. For men, testing previously required a swab to be placed in the urethral meatus; the urine test is easier and less uncomfortable. In addition, several 'near-patient' test kits are available, but these are not validated and may be difficult to use or read.[12]

The new (more expensive) tests make screening for chlamydial infection a more practical proposition, and a national programme is underway.

The National Chlamydia Screening Programme

The plan for a nationwide screening programme was set out in the *National Strategy for Sexual Health and HIV*.[3] The National Chlamydia Screening Programme (NCSP) aims to implement and monitor opportunistic screening for genital *C. trachomatis* infection in young women and men, and in 2004 covered 25% of primary care trusts in England. Ten opportunistic screening programmes were implemented in 2002, and 16 additional programmes were announced in January 2004.[13]

The roll-out programme for the NCSP makes recommendations on screening methods accept-

---

ACTIVITY

Download and read the *Chlamydia Screening Programme Roll-out: Core Requirements*. Available at: http://www.dh.gov.uk

Look at the requirements, and review how your practice manages *Chlamydia* screening.

Undertake an audit of the positive *Chlamydia* results obtained in your practice.

Look at this information in the light of the practice profile and discuss it with your team.

ACTIVITY

Where do you consider is the best place for people to access screening for chlamydial infection?

What are your reasons for this?

Download a copy of the Manual for Sexual Health Advisors available at http://www.ssha.info/public/manual/index.asp (you may wish to keep this on the surgery computer as an electronic resource).

Look at the section on Partner Notification.

Reflect upon the issues of contact tracing and the role of general practice in the management of chlamydial infection.

able to clients. If the client is undergoing a speculum examination, any samples for cervical cytology must be taken before any swabs for *Chlamydia*.[13] If no speculum examination is being carried out, then a self-administered vulval–vaginal swab or (for men and women) a urine sample can be used.[13]

The test manufacturer's instructions should be followed (usually a 'first-catch' urine sample is needed) and the client instructed accordingly. All specimens for the roll-out programme will be tested using nucleic acid amplification tests

(NAATs), to comply with the In-vitro Diagnostic Directive (IVD) (22).[13]

Treatment

Uncomplicated chlamydial infection is simple to treat and cure. The treatment regimens commonly used in the UK are:

- zithromycin 1 g single dose
- oxycycline 100 mg twice daily for 7 days.

Contact tracing should be carried out for all clients with a positive *Chlamydia* result.

CONCLUSION

Changing attitudes to sex have led to a rise in the number of sexually transmitted infections. Chlamydial infection is currently the most common, and it and other STIs can have devastating sequelae if left untreated. Practice nurses are in an ideal position to communicate safer and healthy sex messages to clients.

EVALUATION ACTIVITY

Evaluate how successful any changes have been that you have made to your management of the sexual health of your practice population practice on the basis of what you have learned in this chapter.

LEARNING POINTS

- Contact tracing is an essential component of sexual health services
- GUM clinics occupy a pivotal role, providing the complete range of screening services
- *Chlamydia* currently is the most common STI, particularly among people aged 16–24 years
- The practice nurse is ideally placed to promote sexual health and liase with other services

REFERENCES

1. Adler M, Cowan F, French P, Mitchell H, Richens J. ABC of Sexually Transmitted Infections, 5th edn. London: BMJ Books, 2004.
2. Health Protection Agency. HPA Annual Report and Accounts. Available at: http://www.hpa.org.uk/hpa/publications/ann_rep_2004.htm
3. Department of Health. Better Prevention, Better Services, Better Sexual Health. National Strategy for Sexual Health and HIV. London: HMSO, 2001.
4. Department of Health. Implementation Action Plan. National Strategy for Sexual Health and HIV. London: HMSO, 2002.

5. Society of Sexual Health Advisors. The Manual for Sexual Health Advisors. London: SSHA, 2004. Available at: http://www.ssha.info

6. Dehme K, Snow R. Integrating STI Management into Family Planning Services: What are the Benefits? WHO/RHR/99.10. Geneva: WHO, 1999.

7. Gilson R. Viral hepatitis. In: Adler M, Cowan F, French P, Mitchell H, Richens J (eds), ABC of Sexually Transmitted Infections, 5th edn. London: BMJ Books, 2004.

8. Thomas A, Forster G, Robinson A, Rogstad K. National Guideline on the Management of Suspected Sexually Transmitted Infections in Children and Young People. Available at: http://www.bashh.org/guidelines/2002/adolescent_final_0903.pdf

9. Cowan F. Control and prevention. In: Adler M, Cowan F, French P, Mitchell H, Richens J (eds), ABC of Sexually Transmitted Infections, 5th edn. London: BMJ Books, 2004.

10. French P. The clinical process. In: Adler M, Cowan F, French P, Mitchell H, Richens J (eds), ABC of Sexually Transmitted Infections, 5th edn. London: BMJ Books, 2004.

11. Health Protection Agency. *Chlamydia* Fact Sheet. Available at: http://www.hpa.org.uk/infections/topics_az/hiv_and_sti/sti-chlamydia/general.htm

12. West. Laboratory diagnosis of sexually transmitted infections. In: Adler M, Cowan F, French P, Mitchell H, Richens J (eds), ABC of Sexually Transmitted Infections, 5th edn. London: BMJ Books, 2004.

13. Department of Health. *Chlamydia* Screening Programme Roll-out: Core Requirements. London: HMSO, 2004. Available at: http://www.dh.gov.uk

FURTHER INFORMATION

Adler M, Cowan F, French P, Mitchell H, Richens J (eds). ABC of Sexually Transmitted Infections, 5th edn. London: BMJ Books, 2004.

Health Protection Agency: http://www.hpa.org.uk

Sexual Health Pages: http://www.dh.gov.uk

World Health Organisation: http://www.who.int/health_topics/sexual_health/en

Chapter 16

FEMALE SEXUAL HEALTH

Contraception and unwanted pregnancy I

Sarah Kraszewski

LEARNING OBJECTIVES

After reading this and the following chapter you will be able to:

- evaluate the provision of family planning and sexual health services in your locality and reflect upon how general practice can contribute
- outline the national strategies aimed at reducing the number of teenage and unwanted pregnancies
- understand the categories of contraception available to patients and consider appropriate choices with the patients
- know the routes by which women can access abortion services
- reflect upon the issues of child protection and 'Fraser' competence as applied in the family planning and sexual health context

Attitudes towards sex and sexuality have shifted dramatically over the past 30 years.[1] Issues have emerged to threaten sexual health, but the availability of a broad range of contraceptive methods and sexual health services should enable people to enjoy healthy sex lives (Box 16.1).

This and the following chapter aim to provide an overview of the available methods of contraception and to review the issues of teenage pregnancy and unwanted pregnancy. These two

BOX 16.1   Objectives of the national strategy for sexual health and HIV[1]

- **Reduced** transmission of HIV and sexually transmitted infections (STIs)
- **Lower** rates of unintended pregnancy
- **Reduced** prevalence of undiagnosed human immunodeficiency virus (HIV) and sexually transmitted infections (STIs)
- **Improved** health and social care for people living with HIV
- **Reduction** in the stigma associated with HIV and STIs

BOX 16.2   Defining sexual health[4]

1. **Sexual health is a state of physical, emotional, mental and social well–being related to sexuality;** it is not merely the absence of disease, dysfunction or infirmity

2. **Sexual health requires a positive and respectful approach to sexuality and sexual relationships,** as well as the possibility of having pleasurable and safe sexual experiences, free of coercion, discrimination and violence

3. **For sexual health to be attained and maintained,** the sexual rights of all persons must be respected, protected and fulfilled

chapters should be read bearing in mind the principles of 'Fraser competence'* and with an awareness of potential child protection issues that may arise during the course of sexual health promotion.

Children and young people are entitled to the same duty of confidentiality as adults, providing that individuals aged under 16 years are judged by professionals to understand their choices and the potential outcomes of sharing information [The Fraser Ruling; see Chapter 33, Working with young people, of The Manual for Sexual Health Advisors.[2]]

SEXUAL HEALTH PROMOTION

Sexual health, as defined in Box 16.2, affects the physical and psychological well-being of an individual, and is a central issue in human relationships. It links to the fundamental human rights to privacy, a family life and living free from discrimination.[3]

In recent years, infection rates in the UK for several sexually transmitted infections (STIs) have risen, as have the number of unintended pregnancies (Box 16.3).[1] Improving sexual health entails tackling the issues of ignorance and risky behaviour. Promoting planned parenthood through an

BOX 16.3   Possible consequences of poor sexual health[1]

- Pelvic inflammatory disease, which can cause ectopic pregnancy and infertility
- HIV infection
- Cervical and other genital cancers
- Hepatitis, liver disease and liver cancer
- Recurrent genital herpes
- Bacterial vaginosis and premature delivery
- Unintended pregnancy and subsequent abortion
- Psychological consequences of sexual coercion and abuse
- Poor educational, social and economic opportunities for teenage mothers

Taken from: *Better Prevention, Better Services, Better Sexual Health – The National Strategy for Sexual Health and HIV*, Department of Health, 2001. Available at: http://www.dh.gov.uk

understanding of contraception and how it can be obtained, and increasing the age at which individuals have their first sexual intercourse are important issues in the context of sexual health, and have profound implications in terms of their effect on communities.[1]

General practice offers many opportunities for sexual health promotion. The Royal College of General Practitioners advises that family planning and sexual health services are 'an integral part of primary care' and that general practice should offer 'care and advice on a wide range of sexual matters ... and promote safer sex to all patients'.[5]

ACTIVITY

Obtain a copy of the *Sexual Health Strategy* for your practice from http://www.dh.gov.uk

After reading through the document, identify aspects that relate to the delivery of care in your practice.

METHODS OF CONTRACEPTION

The methods of contraception available in the UK, and their efficacy, are listed in Boxes 16.4 and 16.5.

Combined hormonal contraception

Combined hormonal contraception is the delivery of oestrogen and progestogen on a cyclical basis. The hormones' main mode of action is to prevent ovulation; there are additional effects on the endometrium, cervical mucus and tubal motility.[6] Used correctly, combined hormonal contraception is highly efficacious (around 99%).[7]

A choice of delivery method is now available for combined hormonal contraception: pill or patch. The 'Pill' is presented in 21-day packs, which require a pill-free week between packs, or in 28-day 'everyday' packs; some packs are biphasic or triphasic. The contraceptive patch is a transdermal weekly contraceptive. The user changes the patch weekly for three consecutive weeks, then has a patch-free week. The contra-indications to the use of a combined contraceptive patch are the same as those for the combined oral contraceptive (COC).

BOX 16.4   Available methods of contraception

Combined hormonal contraception
- Combined oral contraceptive pill (COC)
- Combined contraceptive patch

Progestogen–only contraception
- Oral:
  - progestogen-only contraceptive pill (POP)
- Depot:
  - deep intramuscular injection of progestogen (Depo-Provera, Noristerat)
  - subdermal implant of etonogestrel (Implanon)
  - intrauterine system (IUS) of T-shaped intrauterine device and a reservoir of levonorgestrel (Mirena)

Non–hormonal contraceptive devices
- Framed and frameless intrauterine devices (IUDs), inert or copper-bearing

Barrier methods (should be used with a spermicide)
- Male condom
- Female condom
- Diaphragm or cervical cap

Spermicides
- Creams, gels, foams and pessary formulations; used as an adjunct to barrier methods

Natural methods
- Natural family planning

Sterilisation
- Male
- Female

Emergency contraception
- Hormonal methods

Oestrogen–free contraception (OFC)

Progestogen-only contraceptives are available in a variety of formulations and delivery systems. They act chiefly by thickening the cervical mucus,

BOX 16.5   The Pearl Index

The Pearl Index is used to rate the effectiveness of a birth-control method. It refers to the number of unwanted pregnancies in 100 couples using any given method for 1 year. A range of rates is given for each method because:

- long-term users of a method probably have lower pregnancy rates, as those who have failures are likely to change method
- failures are more likely in younger women who may be more fertile and more sexually active

Method	Unwanted pregnancies per 100 couples in first year of use
None (young women)	80–90
None (age 40 years)	40–50
None (age 45 years)	10–20
None (age 50 years)	0–50
Rhythm methods	6–25
Spermicide only	4–25
Coitus interruptus	8–17
Persona fertility device	3–6
Male condom (sheath)	2–15
Female condom	5–15
Diaphragm	4–20
Intrauterine device	0.2–2
Levonorgestrel intrauterine system (IUS)	< 0.5
Progestogen-only pill (POP)	0.3–4
Combined pill (COC)	0.1–3
Subcutaneous implants	0–0.1
Depot medroxyprogesterone injection	0–1
Sterilisation – female	0–0.5
Sterilisation – male	0–0.05

thinning the endometrium and causing some inhibition of ovulation.

The injected formulations suppress ovulation as a primary function. An issue common to all progestogen-only contraceptives is the irregular bleeding pattern or amenorrhoea that may be associated with them; thorough counselling is necessary.

The progestogen-only pill

The progestogen-only pill (POP) is taken continuously, offering efficacy of up to 99% when used correctly.[7] However, there is less margin for error with regard to the timing of doses than with the COC, and the POP demands a high level of concordance.

In addition, factors such as age, lactation and body weight can influence efficacy; some evidence suggests that the POP is less efficacious in women who weigh more than 70 kg.[6] Indications are that desogestrel (Cerazette), a newer POP, inhibits ovulation more successfully and therefore may be more effective than other formulations.[7]

Contraceptive injections

Progestogen-only injections offer effective long-term contraception, users needing to remember only the date their next injection is due. Two types are available. The most widely used is DMPA (depot medroxyprogesterone acetate; Depo-Provera), which provides protection for 12 weeks. An alternative is norethisterone oenanthate (Noristerat), which provides protection for 8 weeks.

The initial injection should be given within the first 5 days of the menstrual cycle, to ensure there is no risk of pregnancy, and if given within this

time it provides immediate cover. The method is fully reversible, but there may be a delay in return to fertility after the last injection, so advice on this is an important part of pre-use counselling.

Contraceptive implants

A small flexible rod containing etonogestrel, placed subcutaneously in the inner upper arm, will provide contraception for 3 years. For women in the UK one implant, Implanon, is available. Implanon is a highly effective contraceptive because, in addition to its inhibition of ovulation, compliance is not an issue – the client cannot forget to take or apply their chosen method.[8] The rod can be removed at any time, with rapid return of fertility to pre-implant status.[8]

Hormonal intrauterine system

The hormonal intrauterine system (IUS) consists of a framed, T-shaped intrauterine device (see below) and a hormone reservoir that is designed to release levonorgestrel daily for up to 5 years.

The device available in the UK is Mirena. The IUS, in common with other progestogen-only methods of contraception, exerts its chief action on the cervical mucus and endometrium; it may inhibit ovulation, but many women using the IUS will continue to ovulate. The method is reversible, with the added advantage that it generally makes periods much lighter and can be used to control menorrhagia.

Careful counselling about the risk of irregular bleeding, particularly during the initial 3 months after insertion, is necessary to enable women to make an informed choice.[6]

Non-hormonal intrauterine devices

An intrauterine device (IUD) is inserted into the uterine cavity for the purpose of preventing pregnancy. IUDs are inserted via the cervical canal and usually contain threads to facilitate removal.[6]

There are framed types, which may be inert, copper-containing or hormone-releasing (see above). There are also frameless devices, which are implanted into the uterus and are copper-bearing or hormonal.[6] An IUD can remain *in situ* and effective for 3–10 years, depending upon the type inserted.

The main effect of an IUD is believed to be the blocking of fertilisation. The inflammatory cells associated with all IUDs impede sperm transport, and the toxic effect of copper on the sperm and ova is also instrumental.[6] Copper IUDs are more effective than inert devices.

EVALUATION ACTIVITY

Reflect critically on the provision of contraceptive services in your area.

How does this serve the client's requirement to access the full range of contraceptives.

ACTIVITY

Consider the advantages and disadvantages of the IUS and IUDs.

For which patients might these methods be particularly suitable?

What availability is there for women in your locality?

Useful information is available in references 6 and 7.

LEARNING POINTS

- The number of unintended pregnancies in the UK has risen in recent years
- Planned parenthood, with an understanding of contraception and how it can be obtained, is of benefit to communities
- A range of effective long-term methods of birth control is available to enable couples to plan and space pregnancies
- Family planning services are an integral part of primary care
- A once-weekly combined hormonal contraceptive patch is now available
- Progestogen injections and contraceptive implants offer effective long-term contraception

---

REFERENCES

1. Department of Health. Better Prevention, Better Services, Better Sexual Health. National Strategy for Sexual Health and HIV. London: HMSO, 2001.
2. Society of Sexual Health Advisors. The Manual for Sexual Health Advisors. London: SSHA, 2004. Available at: http://www.ssha.info
3. House of Commons. Human Rights Act 1998. London: The Stationery Office, 1998.
4. World Health Organisation. Sexual Health. 2002.

Available at: http://www.who.int/reproductive-health/gender/sexual_health.html#3
5. Curtis H, Hoolaghan T, Jewitt C (eds). Sexual Health Promotion in General Practice. Oxford: Radcliffe Medical, 1995.
6. Family Planning Association: http://www.fpa.org.uk
7. Guillebaud J. Contraception: Your Questions Answered, 4th edn. Edinburgh: Churchill Livingstone, 2004.

8. Organon International. Implanon (etonogestrel). Available at: http://www.organon.com/products/ contraception/Implanon.asp?ComponentID= 10125&SourcePageID=53906

FURTHER INFORMATION

British Pregnancy Advisory Service: charitable organisation for women and girls who need advice on issues relating to pregnancy, emergency contraception and abortion. http://www.bpas.org

Department of Health: a range of sexual health resources for healthcare professionals. http://www.dh.gov.uk/ PolicyAndGuidance/HealthAndSocialCareTopics/ SexualHealth/fs/en

Faculty of Family Planning and Reproductive Health Care (part of the Royal College of Obstetricians & Gynaecologists): the website provides information on training courses, meetings, guidelines and publications. http://www.ffprhc.org.uk

fpa (formerly known as the Family Planning Association): a registered charity that aims to improve the sexual health and reproductive rights of all people throughout the UK, working with the public and professionals to ensure high-quality information and services are available to everyone who needs them. http://www.fpa.org.uk

Health Protection Agency: HIV and sexually transmitted infections; epidemiological data, reports, guidelines and publications. http://www.hpa.org.uk/infections/topics_az/ hiv_and_sti/publications/annual2004/annual2004.htm

Marie Stopes International UK: the country's leading reproductive healthcare charity, helping over 70,000 women and men each year. http://www.mariestopes.org.uk

Playing Safely: the NHS guide to the symptoms, treatment and prevention of sexually transmitted infections (STIs) and diseases (STDs), including *Chlamydia*, genital warts, herpes, syphilis and gonorrhoea. http://www.playingsafely.co.uk

RCN Distance Learning Course: Royal College of Nursing course in sexual health skills. For details visit: http://www.rcn.org.uk/resources/sexualhealth; or e-mail sexualhealthPND@rcn.org.uk

Teenage Pregnancy Unit: information about the Government's Teenage Pregnancy Strategy. There is also information about local implementation of the strategy and details about the Independent Advisory Group on Teenage Pregnancy. http://www.dfes.gov.uk/teenagepregnancy

Chapter 17

FEMALE SEXUAL HEALTH

Contraception and unwanted pregnancy II

Sarah Kraszewski

LEARNING OBJECTIVES

After reading this and the previous chapter you will be able to:

- evaluate the provision of family planning and sexual health services in your locality and reflect upon how general practice can contribute
- outline the national strategies aimed at reducing the number of teenage and unwanted pregnancies
- understand the categories of contraception available to clients and consider appropriate choices with the clients
- know the routes by which women can access abortion services
- reflect upon the issues of child protection and 'Fraser' competence as applied in the family planning and sexual health context

Issues relating to sexual health, including the practice nurse's role in sexual health promotion, and methods of contraception are discussed in Chapter 16. This chapter looks at barrier methods of contraception, natural family planning, sterilisation and emergency contraception. It concludes with a discussion of teenage and unwanted pregnancies.

BARRIER METHODS OF CONTRACEPTION

Barrier methods of contraception present a physical barrier to prevent sperm from entering the uterine cavity. They have an additional important role in promoting safer sex for all ages, as they may help prevent the transmission of sexually transmitted infections (STIs).

Condoms

Male and female condoms are available. Male condoms (sheaths) are manufactured from latex or polyurethane and are available in a variety of fittings, finishes, colours and flavours, and with various lubricants. Female condoms are manufactured from polyurethane.

The efficacy of a condom will depend entirely upon the users. Common problems include failure to put a condom on before sexual contact, the male condom falling off, and damage to the condom (e.g. from the use of oil-based lubricants or splits and tears caused by fingernails or jewellery). Female condoms may get pushed into the vagina, or the penis may be inserted outside the condom.

Diaphragms and caps

Diaphragms and caps are placed inside the vagina to cover the cervix. Diaphragms are circular domes of thin rubber, about 55–100 mm in diameter, and are available with a variety of flexible metal rims or springs. Cervical caps are smaller, about 20–30 mm in diameter, and stay in place by suction; newer silicone varieties are becoming available.[1]

Diaphragms and caps should always be used with a spermicide, and additional spermicide used for repeated intercourse. A nurse or doctor trained in family planning should carry out the initial fitting of diaphragms and caps, and teach the patient how to use them correctly. A fitting check should be carried out every 6–12 months; re-fitting is required if the woman's weight varies by more than 3.5 kg and following pregnancy.

NATURAL FAMILY PLANNING

Natural family planning (NFP) or fertility awareness enables women to recognise fertile and infertile times during the menstrual cycle and thus time intercourse to achieve or avoid pregnancy. There are three main ways to determine when ovulation is likely. These are:

- the calendar method (a woman's fertile period is 12–16 days before her period starts)
- the temperature method (a woman's temperature, measured on waking, will go up by about 0.5°C the day after ovulation, under the influence of progesterone)
- mucus test (the mucus produced by a woman's vagina and cervix changes in character during her cycle, reflecting fluctuating levels of oestrogen and progesterone).

If a woman's cycle is irregular, it is more difficult to predict when ovulation is likely. Women wishing to use fertility awareness methods to avoid pregnancy should consult an NFP teacher. The fpa can provide further information.

Breastfeeding

While a baby is under 6 months old and fully breastfed, and the mother has amenorrhoea, breastfeeding may be used as a natural method of contraception; however, all three conditions must apply.[1]

Fertility devices

The variation of hormone levels in a woman's urine during the menstrual cycle is another indicator of times when she is fertile. The main device available in the UK to utilise this variation is Persona. If a woman tests the hormone levels in her urine at particular times in her cycle, the device will predict fertile and infertile times. It is not available on prescription. Used according to instructions it is 94% effective.[1]

Female and male sterilisation

The option of sterilisation for one or both sexual partners is an effective way to prevent ova and sperm meeting. However, although this method of contraception has become increasingly popular, it should be considered only for people who are sure they never want children or whose families are complete.

The male and female procedures entail occlusion of the vas deferens (hence, vasectomy) or the fallopian tubes, respectively, and must be regarded as permanent. Reversal carries no guarantee of success, and may not be available on the NHS.

In 2004 the Royal College of Obstetricians and Gynaecologists issued updated guidelines on male and female sterilisation.[2] The role of the procedure in family planning will need to be reconsidered as other long-term but reversible contraceptive options become available.

EMERGENCY CONTRACEPTION

If a couple's chosen method of contraception fails or if a woman has unprotected sexual intercourse, the woman may obtain one of two types of emergency contraception.

The hormonal method of emergency contraception requires the woman to take one tablet of levonorgestrel 1500 µg up to 72 hours after unprotected intercourse. The sooner after unprotected intercourse the dose is taken, the more likely it is to prevent conception. The intended action of the pills is to stop or delay ovulation and prevent implantation.

Alternatively, the woman can have inserted a copper-bearing intrauterine device (IUD), the aim of which is to prevent implantation. This is the most efficacious method of emergency contraception, and the device may be inserted up to 5 days after unprotected intercourse.

ACTIVITY

Clarify the key issues that need to be addressed at a consultation for emergency contraception.

How do clients in your locality access emergency contraception when the GP surgery is closed?

What arrangements are there in your locality for under-16s to access emergency contraception?

How might you work collaboratively with other professionals (such as school nurses) to develop services?

Review the issue of consent in the under-16s ('Fraser' competence). A useful resource is *Reference Guide to Consent for Examination or Treatment*, Department of Health, 2001. Available at: http://www.dh.gov.uk

Consider the child protection issues this might raise. How would you approach a consultation where you felt there might be child protection issues to broach?

TEENAGE PREGNANCY

England's teenage birth rates are the highest in western Europe.[3] One in every ten babies born in England has a teenage mother, who is more likely to have a poor background than to belong, say, to a professional family. The children of teenage mothers have an increased risk of growing up in disadvantaged circumstances, with poor health and social outcomes. For example, infant mortality rates for babies born to mothers below 18 years of age are twice the national average.[4]

A report from the Social Exclusion Unit (SEU) on teenage pregnancy in 1999 proposed an integrated strategy to tackle the problems and social exclusion issues raised by teenage pregnancy. The report sets out a 10-year strategy, based on a 30-point action plan. The broad themes are:

- 'joined up' action at local and national level
- a national campaign to support young people in making their own choices and taking responsibility for their actions
- better teaching on sex and relationships
- better access to contraceptive advice
- better support for pregnant teenagers and teenage parents, to increase their access to and participation in education, training and employment, and thus reduce the risks of social exclusion.

In March 2004, the Teenage Pregnancy Unit reported that the 30-point strategy is being implemented in full, with consequent reported reductions in conception rates (Box 17.1).[5]

Sure Start Plus, an initiative to support pregnant teenagers and teenage parents under 18 years old, was launched in April 2001. A 5-year pilot study is being carried out at 20 sites around England covering 35 local authority areas. The aims are to improve health, education and social outcomes for teenagers who are pregnant or who are already parents, and for their children.

Sure Start Plus and Connexions, the Government support service for young people aged 13–19 years in England, work collaboratively to

---

BOX 17.1   The teenage pregnancy strategy for England

Aims set out in 1999[4]
- Reduce the rate of teenage conceptions. The specific aim is to halve the rate of conceptions among those under 18 years by 2010, with an interim reduction of 15% by 2004
- Achieve a firmly established downward trend in conception rates in those under 16 years by 2010
- Increase the participation of teenage parents in education and work, to reduce their risk of long-term social exclusion

Progress report, March 2004[5]
- Conceptions in teenagers aged under 18 years: 9.4% reduction between 1998 and 2002
- Conceptions in teenagers aged under 16 years: 11% reduction since 2001
- Proportion of teenage parents in education and training or work: 26.3% in 2003, compared with 16% in 1997

ACTIVITY

What family planning services are available for young people in your area?

In particular, how can a young person under the age of 16 years access free emergency contraception?

ACTIVITY

Visit the Teenage Pregnancy Unit website, and review the aims of the National Teenage Pregnancy Strategy and the work of agencies such as Sure Start Plus and Connexions. http://www.dfes.gov.uk/teenagepregnancy

Find out what initiatives are operating in your locality.

Consider how general practice can contribute to the aims of the National Teenage Pregnancy Strategy.

contribute to the aims of the National Teenage Pregnancy Strategy, and engage with other agencies.[5]

UNWANTED PREGNANCY

Unwanted pregnancy may be diagnosed in a variety of settings, such as general practice, a family planning or genitourinary medicine (GUM) clinic or the client's home, but wherever the diagnosis is made it is a distressing experience for the woman involved.[6] The upset is quickly followed by a need for complex decision-making and the health professional's role is to support the client through the discovery, and to clarify the options available to her, while working within the various legal and ethical frameworks.[7–10]

Of paramount concern are the needs of the client,[7] who must be allowed time to consider all the options and make an informed decision. The immediate reaction of some women is to accede to the demands of others, rather than give precedence to their own needs.[7] The role of the health professional in this consultation is to support the client, who needs to work out her own wishes with regard to the pregnancy and decide on the appropriate action. The client needs also to take responsibility for that decision and to realise how she came to be in the situation, and know how to avoid it recurring.[11]

WHAT ARE THE OPTIONS?

Three choices exist for the woman who has an unwanted pregnancy. She may opt to continue the pregnancy and keep the baby. This decision will have life-changing consequences, and raises issues such as the requirement for antenatal care and family and social support. An alternative is to continue the pregnancy but have the baby adopted, in which case antenatal care will again be required, together with pre-adoption coun-

selling to ensure the woman understands her choice. The woman's third option is to request termination of her pregnancy.

Termination of pregnancy

Women wishing referral for an NHS-funded abortion should visit their GP, a family or young persons' clinic, or a GUM/sexual health or walk-in clinic. Those preferring to seek a privately funded abortion can refer themselves to an approved independent-sector provider, through a registered pregnancy advice bureau or a registered medical practitioner.[12]

BOX 17.2 Circumstances under which an abortion may be performed (The Abortion Act 1967, amended 1990)

Two registered medical practitioners, acting in good faith, must agree that the pregnancy should be terminated on one or more of the following grounds:

- The risk to the woman's life is greater if the pregnancy is continued than if the pregnancy is terminated
- The termination will prevent serious, permanent injury to the physical or mental health of the pregnant woman
- Gestation is no more than 24 weeks, and there is greater risk of injury to the physical or mental health of the pregnant woman if the pregnancy is continued than if it is terminated
- Gestation is no more than 24 weeks, and there is greater risk of injury to the physical or mental health of the existing children of the family if the pregnancy is continued than if it is terminated
- There is substantial risk that at birth this child would have physical or mental abnormalities causing a serious handicap or special need

The Abortion Act (1967, amended 1990) defines in law the specific circumstances under which an abortion may be performed (Box 17.2). This Act does not apply to Northern Ireland.[13]

The World Health Organization estimates that around 40–50 million abortions are carried out each year. Every day, tens of thousands of women around the world are having to make what is probably one of the most difficult decisions of their lives.[14] When, following support and counselling, a woman decides to request an abortion, a referral should be activated without delay. The National Strategy for Sexual Health and HIV sets a waiting time target of 3 weeks from first appointment to abortion for women who meet the legal criteria.[1]

METHODS OF ABORTION

There are several methods of abortion and local availability will vary. Within the first trimester, a medical abortion may be offered. Mifepristone (Mifegyne) 600 mg is given as a single dose orally. This is followed after 48 hours with gemeprost 1 mg, administered per vagina, following which the uterus contracts to expel the fetus within 4 hours.[15] The Royal College of Obstetricians and Gynaecologists guidelines for early medical abortions also recommend the unlicensed use of mifepristone 200 mg orally followed 1–3 days later by misoprostol 800 μg vaginally. If abortion has not occurred after 4 hours in women with gestation of 49–63 days, a further dose of misoprostol may be give orally or per vagina.[16]

Vacuum aspiration may be carried out up to 14 weeks' gestation,[7] under conscious sedation or general anaesthetic. Beyond 14 weeks, abortion has more complications, and may be medical or surgical depending upon the opinion of the gynaecologist.

Following a termination of pregnancy, a health professional must address the woman's future contraceptive needs, and advise her how to access contraceptive supplies. Also, the availability needs to be established of post-termination support services, in order to enable women to explore their feelings of grief and loss following this event.[6]

CONCLUSION

Family planning services are an integral part of primary care, and the practice nurse can play a

LEARNING POINTS

- Sexual health promotion requires a knowledge of the availability and suitability of different forms of contraception
- The practice nurse needs to be aware of how her patients can access local sexual health services
- Teenage pregnancy can adversely affect the social, psychological and physical health of mother and child
- Unwanted pregnancy is distressing, and health professionals need to be able to support unhappily pregnant women in making what is the right decision for them about how to proceed

key part in promoting planned parenthood and offering support in the event of unwanted pregnancy.

EVALUATION ACTIVITY

Reflect critically on the access to services for women with unwanted pregnancy.

Identify the client pathway.

REFERENCES

1. fpa (formerly the Family Planning Association): http://www.fpa.org.uk
2. Royal College of Obstetricians and Gynaecologists. Male and Female Sterilisation: Guideline Summary. Evidence-based Clinical Guideline 4. London: RCOG, 2004. Available at: http://www.rcog.org.uk
3. Department of Health. Better Prevention, Better Services, Better Sexual Health. National Strategy for Sexual Health and HIV. London: The Stationery Office, 2001.
4. Department of Health. Government Response to the First Annual Report of the Independent Advisory Group on Teenage Pregnancy. London: The Stationery Office, 2002.
5. Teenage Pregnancy Unit. Implementation of the Teenage Pregnancy Strategy: Progress Report. Available at: http://www.dfes.gov.uk/teenagepregnancy
6. Davies V. Abortion and Afterwards. Bath: Ashgrove Press, 1991.
7. Society of Sexual Health Advisors. The Manual for Sexual Health Advisors. London: SSHA, 2004. Available at: http://www.ssha.info
8. Family Planning Association. Abortion: Legal and Ethical Issues. Fact File 6B. London: fpa.
9. House of Commons. 1998 Human Rights Act. London: The Stationery Office, 1998.
10. Department of Health. Guidelines for Implementing the 1967 Abortion Act. Health Circular (77) 26. London: HMSO, 1967.
11. Filshie M. Termination of pregnancy. In: Louden N (ed.), Handbook of Family Planning. Edinburgh: Churchill Livingstone, 1991.
12. Department of Health. Pregnancy Advice Bureaux. Available at: http://www.dh.gov.uk/PolicyAndGuidance/HealthandSocialCareTopics/SexualHealth
13. House of Commons. 1967 Abortion Act. London: HMSO, 1967.
14. World Health Organization. Safe Abortion: Technical and Policy Guidance for Health Systems. Geneva: WHO, 2003.
15. GP Notebook. http://www.gpnotebook.co.uk
16. Royal College of Obstetricians and Gynaecologists. The Care of Women Requesting Induced Abortion. Evidence-based Clinical Guideline No. 7. London: RCOG, 2004. Available at: http://www.rcog.org.uk

Chapter 18

FEMALE SEXUAL HEALTH
Female sexual dysfunction

Tina Bishop

LEARNING OBJECTIVES

After reading this chapter you will be able to:

- identify a range of problems that may affect female sexual function
- discuss myths and misconceptions that affect beliefs and attitudes to female sexual disorders
- understand the nature and causes of female sexual dysfunction
- outline an appropriate response when working with a client who identifies a specific sexual dysfunction

We do not have much information on the nature and prevalence of sexual problems in people attending general practice, but in one UK study 41% of women and 34% of men admitted to problems with sexual function.[1] It is only in the past 10 years or so that female sexual dysfunction has been recognised, investigated and treated by the medical profession, and the existence acknowledged of physical and psychological problems that might need to be addressed.

In the promotion of sexual health and well-being, the focus is usually on contraceptive advice, healthy pregnancy and the avoidance of sexually transmitted infections. However, sexual health is about much more than medical matters. Integral to sexual health are the ideas, views and feelings (Box 18.1) that we have about our own and others' sexuality.[2]

CHANGING ATTITUDES

Commonly held views on issues relating to women and sexuality have changed radically. In the past, women were seen as passive, non-sexual beings and sexual intercourse was a means to an end, the woman's role being solely the procreation of children. Today, sexual expression is accepted as a source of pleasure and fulfilment for both men and women, although notions of what is 'normal' sexual activity are many and varied. In this respect, women differ greatly one from another, and will also experience change throughout their lives. Moreover, expectations of sexual activity for men and women may be different, and the idea persists that men are always ready for sex but women may be frigid. It seems that many people think the norm to be sexual activity that always results in full penetrative sexual intercourse with orgasm, but loving, fulfilling relationships between couples may not always depend on sexual intercourse.

MAKING A DIFFERENCE

Practice nurses are in an ideal position to address many of the challenges raised by female sexual dysfunction. From health promotion and dispelling myths to giving advice and making referrals, there are many opportunities to make a real difference to women's sexual health and well-being. Many GPs and practice nurses have a special interest in sexual health and have taken further training to support their role in the practice. Not all practice nurses can be expected to possess specialist knowledge and skills in this area; however, it is important to be aware of the range of sexual problems with which women may present, and to understand the common

---

BOX 18.1   Feelings that adversely affect a woman's sexuality[2]

Misunderstandings about sex
- Ignorance about sex
- Not knowing what to expect
- Not knowing how to behave
- Expectations too high

Bad feelings about sex
- Fear of being caught
- Fear of making too much noise and being overheard
- Fear of being interrupted
- Fear of failing to perform 'normally'
- Fear of being undignified or incontinent
- Guilt, belief that sexual intercourse or sexual acts are wrong
- Disgust that sex is dirty and messy

Problems in the relationship
- Feeling angry, even rage and violence
- Feeling resentful and bitter
- Feeling contempt for a partner
- Feeling insecure
- Fear of being physically hurt
- Fear of partner leaving
- Fear of the future

Bad feelings about oneself
- Depression
- Worthlessness
- Low self-esteem
- Unattractive
- Unhappy with her body image

Circumstances that cause lack of sexual feelings
- Too tired
- Worried
- Preoccupied with other things
- Babies and children of all ages
- Lack of warmth and comfort
- Losses and bereavement
- No privacy

---

treatments and management approaches and whom to refer.

Think about the term 'female sexual dysfunction'. What does it mean to you? What might it mean to a patient?

What are the kinds of problem that fall under this umbrella term?

FEMALE SEXUAL DYSFUNCTION: WHAT DOES IT ENCOMPASS?

Female sexual dysfunction is a term used to describe problems with a woman's sex life that cause her distress. Anxieties around sexual orientation or variation of sexual practice are not classed as sexual dysfunction, although they may affect sexual function. There are many reasons why women may experience problems with their sex life, which might include medical conditions, medication and life experience (Table 18.1).

There is a general classification used to describe female sexual difficulties and anxieties (Box 18.2), which provides a framework for defining and treating them, and each category is discussed here in turn. Dysfunction can also be further classified as primary, where problems have been present since the start of sexual activity, or secondary, where problems develop after a period of satisfactory sexual function.

Inhibited desire

Sex drive is the biological factor that makes women think about sex and behave sexually. There are many reasons why women may experience low sex drive; it can be a physical

TABLE 18.1   Common causes of sexual dysfunction

Cause type	Dysfunction type		
	Decreased sexual desire	Problems with arousal	Problems with orgasm
Medical conditions	• Serious or chronic illness • Central nervous system (CNS) disease	• Vascular disease • Menopause • Diabetes • Alcoholism	• Diabetes • Vascular disease • Chronic illness
Medications	• Antipsychotic drugs • Phenothiazines • Butyrophenones, e.g. haloperidol • Cimetidine and other antihistamines • Narcotics • Tricyclic antidepressants • SSRIs • Antihistamines • Anticholinergic • Beta blockers	• Beta blockers • Thiazide diuretics • ACE inhibitors • CNS-active drugs • Antihypertensives • Antihistamines • Benzodiazepines	• Narcotics • Sedatives • Alcohol • Tricyclic antidepressants • SSRIs • Benzodiazepines
Life experiences	• Sexual trauma, rape, abuse • Depression, anger and difficulties in relationships • Negative body image • Chronic stress • Fatigue	• Stress • Fatigue • Anxiety • Inadequate stimulation	• Inadequate stimulation • Fear of loss of control • Lack of knowledge

BOX 18.2   Classification of female sexual dysfunction[4]

- Inhibited desire disorder: lack of, or loss of interest in, sexual desire
- Sexual arousal disorder: persistent or recurrent absence of sexual arousal
- Sexual pain disorder: painful intercourse
- Orgasmic dysfunction: difficulty achieving, or absence of, orgasm

problem, a psychological problem or a combination of both. Tiredness, depression and illness can affect a woman's energy levels and sexual desire, for example a woman who has recently given birth or had an operation may experience a temporary loss of interest in sex, while for others there may be a physical cause such as diabetes or hypertension. There may also be relationship problems, alone or in combination with any of the above.

Sexual arousal disorder

During sexual arousal several physical responses take place that make penetration comfortable. The clitoris becomes engorged with blood and swells in size. The tissues that surround the entrance to the vagina open slightly, and there is an increase in vaginal lubrication. Clearly, if intercourse were to take place without this response, the experience would be at least uncomfortable or possibly painful, and could lead to further anxieties for the future. Sexual arousal is a vascular event, and any physical problem that interferes with this response can contribute to the problem.

Sexual pain disorder

Community studies undertaken in the UK in the late 1990s found that 18% of women experienced pain during intercourse (dyspareunia), and comparable studies in the USA revealed similar numbers.[1, 5] There are three types of dyspareunia:

- insertional pain
- pain in a specific area of the vulva or vagina
- pain with deep penetration.

The causes are listed in Box 18.3.

Vaginismus

A condition that makes penetration almost impossible is vaginismus, which is involuntary spasm of the muscle around the opening of the vagina. This condition is a major cause of non-consummation of marriage.

BOX 18.3   Causes of dyspareunia[3]

Insertional dyspareunia
- Lubrication difficulties:
  - lack of knowledge of sexual response
  - lack of arousal
  - postmenopausal atrophy
- Vulvitis – infectious or irritative
- Vaginitis – infectious or irritative
- Vaginismus
- Psychological concerns

Pain in a specific area of the vulva or vagina
- Hymenal ring difficulty
- Old scars, lesions, abscesses, gland enlargement
- Vulvitis – infectious or irritative
- Vaginitis – infectious or irritative

Pain with deep penetration
- Masses or uterine enlargement
- Endometriosis
- Adhesions
- Vaginismus
- Condyloma acuminata (genital warts)
- Psychological concerns

Orgasmic disorder

Some women, even though their sexual responsiveness is normal, may not achieve an orgasm, and this may be disappointing for both the woman and her partner. Reasons for not experiencing an orgasm range from a lack of arousal to a lack of stimulation from a partner, and other factors may include poor housing or lack of privacy.

ACTIVITY

Consider your work base. Is there information about female sexual dysfunction available for patients to read and take away?

Is it clear and easy to read?

Where is the information placed?

Could it be better displayed, or positioned in such a way that it can be read or gathered without others observing?

RESPONDING TO A FEMALE PATIENT WITH A SEXUAL DYSFUNCTION: ROLE OF THE PRACTICE NURSE

Taking a history

A detailed medical and sexual history should be obtained from all women who are distressed or unhappy with any aspect of their sexual health. A vaginal examination, with the patient's permission, may be required.

Investigations might include a blood test to check hormone levels; a urine test and blood pressure check would also be relevant to exclude diabetes and hypertension. Treatment of any medical condition that might be contributing to the problem should always be tackled first.

Sensitive interviewing and communication skills are required; women may find it difficult and embarrassing to discuss aspects of their private lives with a doctor or nurse. As Dr Gill has commented, 'The private parts are not so-called for nothing'.[6]

Practice nurses already have consultations with patients, such as taking a cervical smear, that involve undertaking an intimate examination. A patient could choose this time to mention to you their fears or problems or ask advice. You might feel 'out of your depth' when sensitive information is confided to you, and be unable to offer a solution. It is important that you do not feel you have to. Being open, non-judgmental and able to listen, and asking the patient's permission to share their concerns with the most appropriate member of staff, may be the extent of your role in helping the patient.

ACTIVITY

Think about a situation when you have been asked, or when you might be asked, for advice about female sexual dysfunction.

How did or do you feel about this?

What factors will determine the success of your contribution in such instances?

Treatment

Treatment of sexual dysfunction depends on accurate diagnosis. One or more problems may coexist and it is easy to see how one problem can lead to another.

There are different types of treatments and patients may need one or a combination of the following:

- medical treatment
- lifestyle advice/management (e.g. obesity, alcohol consumption)
- psychosexual therapy
- counselling.

It is beyond the scope of this chapter to list all possible treatments, but the management of vaginismus provides an example of combination therapy. Treatment is usually based on sex education, psychological counselling and use of vaginal trainers. Vaginal trainers are plastic, dome-shaped devices that come in four graduated sizes. The woman uses the smallest trainer first, inserted into the vagina, and when that is comfortable the next size is used. Use of the trainers is combined with psychological counsell-ing that aims to explore with the patient her knowledge and understanding, and anxieties and feelings around sex and sexual activity. The treatment is centred on each individual woman, who plays an active part in her own treatment. The doctor/psychotherapist facilitates the treatment plan until the patient is comfortable with her sexual feelings and activities.

relaxing the blood vessels in the penis and thereby aid erection. Viagra is under investigation for use in women, and there are conflicting reports of benefits. Some criticism has been voiced of the pharmaceutical industry because their activities can be seen as 'building the science of female dysfunction'.[8]

For most people, a good sex life is an important part of what makes them happy. Doctors and nurses working in general practice need to be alert to patients consulting with sexual problems. The recognition and management of sexual dysfunction is an area that presents health professionals with many challenges, and might identify training and management issues above and beyond providing the usual contraceptive health advice.

ACTIVITY

Identify the resources available in your area to support women with sexual dysfunction.

Is there a GP or practice nurse with a special interest in this subject? Are there local clinics? Who runs the services?

Discuss with your colleagues which resources are available and make your own list of them.

EVALUATION ACTIVITY

On the basis of what you have learned from this chapter, evaluate the success of any changes you have made to practice.

CONCLUSION

In 2003 in a study set in 13 London general practices, 21% of men and 30% of women reported seeking sexual advice from their GP.[7] The study concluded that sexual difficulties are common in the practice population and that patients are prepared to discuss them with their doctor.

Sexual dysfunction in men appears to have a higher public profile than that in women, mainly as a result of the identification of erectile dysfunction and the development of oral pharmaceutical treatments such as Viagra (sildenafil). These drugs are not aphrodisiacs; they are phosphodiesterase type 5 drugs that work by

---

LEARNING POINTS

- Sexual difficulties are common, and many women will experience one at some point in their lives
- Sexual dysfunction is difficulty engaging in, or inability to engage in, sexual activity, which arises from a physical or psychological disorder or a combination of both. This does not include variations in sexual practices or sexual orientation
- If you are uncomfortable discussing sexual problems, refer patients to others until you have had sufficient opportunity to observe, develop and refine your skills
- Sexual difficulties are common in people attending general practice and many patients are willing to talk about them

REFERENCES

1. Dunn KM, Croft PR, Hackett GI. Sexual problems: a study of the prevalence and need for health care in the general population. Family Practice 1998; 15: 519–524.
2. Selby J. Psychosexual and emotional care. In: Andrew G (ed.), Women's Sexual Health, 2nd edn. London: Harcourt, 2001.
3. Lenahan P, Ellwood A. Sexuality and sexual dysfunction through the life cycle. In: Rosenfeld J (ed.), A Handbook of Women's Health. Cambridge: Cambridge University Press, 2001.
4. Basson R, Berman J, Burnett A, et al. Report on the international consensus development conference on female sexual dysfunction; definitions of classifications. J Urology 2000; 163: 888–893.
5. Laumann EO, Paik A, Rosen RC. Sexual dysfunction in the United States: prevalence and predictors. JAMA 1999; 281: 537–544.
6. Gill M. Defences in the patient. In: Skrine R (ed.), Introductions to Psychosexual Medicine. London: Chapman & Hall, 1989.
7. Nazareth I, Boynton P, King M. Problems with sexual function in people attending London general practitioners: cross sectional study. BMJ 2003; 327: 423.
8. Moynihan R. The making of a disease: female sexual dysfunction. BMJ 2003; 236: 45–47.

FURTHER INFORMATION

British Association of Sexual and Relationship Therapy: a national charity whose website provides a list of therapists, links to related organisations, information for the general public and password-protected information for members. http://www.basrt.org.uk

Relate: a charity that offers advice, relationship counselling, sex therapy, workshops, mediation, and support. Help is available face to face, by phone and online through the website. Relateline: 0845 130 4010; http://www.relate.org.uk/sexproblems

Sexual Dysfunction Association: a registered charity that provides information on various conditions affecting sexual function. Tel. 0870 7743571; http://www.sda.uk.net

Chapter 19

MALE SEXUAL HEALTH
Male sexual dysfunction

Graham Harris

LEARNING OBJECTIVES

After reading this chapter you will be able to:

- identify a range of problems that may affect male sexual function
- discuss myths and misconceptions that affect beliefs and attitudes to male sexual disorders
- understand the nature and causes of erectile dysfunction
- discuss strategies that can help to minimise or overcome problems associated with erectile dysfunction
- outline an appropriate response when working with a client who identifies a specific sexual dysfunction

As a topic, sexual dysfunction tends to be something of a conversation stopper – a brief mention is often enough to generate uncomfortable coughs, embarrassed laughs and even a sudden search for coats and car keys.[1] Men, in particular, seem to find this a difficult area, and are often reticent to share their concerns about such matters.[2, 3] Yet sexual difficulties are so common that almost all men will experience one at some point in their lives,[4–6] and suffering in silence is pointless because much can be done to help.

Practice nurses are in an ideal position to address many of the challenges raised by male sexual dysfunction. From health promotion and dispelling myths to giving advice and making referrals, there are many opportunities to make a real difference to men's sexual health and well-being. Not all practice nurses can be expected to possess specialist knowledge and skills in this area, but it is important to be aware of the range of sexual problems with which men may present, and to understand the common treatments and management approaches.

ACTIVITY

Think about the term 'male sexual dysfunction'.

What does it mean to you?

What might it mean to a patient?

What problems fall under this umbrella term?

MALE SEXUAL DYSFUNCTION: EXPLORING THE TERRITORY

The term 'male sexual dysfunction' may conjure up all manner of ideas and images, but what does the term actually mean? Quite simply, sexual dysfunction is difficulty engaging in, or inability to engage in, sexual activity, which arises from a physical or psychological disorder or a combination of both. This does not include variations in sexual practices or sexual orientation; anxiety about either of these can affect sexual function but they are not sexual dysfunctions in themselves, and should not be treated as such.

The problems encountered range from mild, transient difficulties to major, long-term disorders. They can also be considered in terms of the stages of the male sexual response (Table 19.1), in particular the first three stages: desire, arousal and ejaculation.

Problems with desire

Three problems experienced in relation to desire are:

- excessive desire (sometimes known as sex addiction)
- a loss or lack of desire (sometimes known as loss of libido)
- being 'out of synch' with a partner, as a consequence of either of the above.

This chapter deals with the first and last of these problems. Excessive desire does not seem to be common and the related literature is sparse; in such instances men can usually be referred to an appropriate sex therapist.

If a man's desire for sexual activity is greater or less than his partner's, this can cause major tensions in the relationship, and such problems are likely to be referred on, possibly for couple counselling.

The problem of loss of desire warrants a little more discussion, mainly because it is not usually thought of as a male problem. Although myth suggests that men are always ready for and wanting sex, the reality is that 'going off it' is not

TABLE 19.1 Stages in the male sexual response[7]	
Stage	Definition
Desire	The wish to engage in sexual activity, triggered by thoughts and verbal, visual or other cues
Arousal	The state of sexual excitement that occurs as blood enters the genital area (leading to erection)
Orgasm	The climax of sexual excitement that occurs at ejaculation, with increased muscle tension throughout the body
Resolution	The sense of well-being and muscle relaxation that follows orgasm

uncommon, and occurs for many different reasons. Tiredness, boredom and stress outside of the relationship need to be considered. So too do worries, such as the risk of making a partner pregnant or failing to live up to a partner's expectations. The fear of failure is especially important because it can ultimately turn a man off sex, so he will avoid it altogether and thus set up a vicious circle that maintains the problem.[3, 4]

However, a loss of desire or reduced libido must not be dismissed as a mainly psychological problem. Heavy drinking and the use of drugs may play a part, and in medical conditions, such as liver or heart disease or rheumatoid arthritis, reduced libido can be just one of many symptoms. In fact, any health condition can reduce libido, as can many medications. Hence, in all cases, assessment needs to be thorough, and followed by appropriate referral.

Problems with arousal

The most common of the many problems associated with arousal in men (Box 19.1) is erectile dysfunction, or male erectile disorder (the term 'impotence' is no longer used).[4]

Most definitions of the condition refer to a persistent inability to attain or sustain an erection sufficiently rigid to allow satisfactory sexual performance.[8–11] The range of dysfunction is wide, from men who can no longer get an erection at all to those who achieve one but can sustain it for only a few minutes. So why does it happen?

Until the mid-1980s, most experts insisted that 90% of erection problems were purely psychological.[4] Today, most suggest the reverse: that around 10–20% of cases are psychological, and the rest physical or caused by a combination of physical and psychological factors.[6, 9–11]

Physical problems

Most physical causes are related to the circulatory or neurological systems. Less common physical causes include hormonal abnormalities, alcoholism and drug abuse

Circulatory problems affecting blood flow to the penis may occur in hypertension, diabetes mellitus and cardiac disease, where there is poor vascularity because of atherosclerosis or arteriosclerosis. It is not only the blood supply to the penis that is important though, as drainage of blood from the penis is also critical; in some men, vein injury or disease leads to excessive drainage or 'venous leak'.[4, 7]

Neurological problems affecting penile erection can arise from conditions such as multiple sclerosis, spinal injury and, again, diabetes mellitus. Parkinson's disease and Alzheimer's disease may be responsible.[7] Neuroimpairment may also arise as a consequence of surgery or radiotherapy to the pelvic area.

A drug and medication history is important, because erection problems may well occur as a side-effect of treatment, a good example being antihypertensive medications.

Psychological problems

Psychological causes of erectile dysfunction include some of those mentioned for loss of libido: anxiety, fear of failure and stress in other areas of life. 'Performance angst' is a significant factor, sometimes born of an excessive wish to please a partner. Certain situations and specific circumstances can similarly create difficulties; in cramped conditions or where there is the possibility of being observed, some men find their anxieties become all-consuming.

Age

Although most cases of erectile dysfunction occur in men over 40 years old, it must be made clear that ageing does not cause erectile dysfunction. Ageing may bring changes (Box 19.2), but there is no reason why older men should not enjoy, and indeed expect to enjoy, fulfilling sexual lives.[11, 12] Sadly, research from the USA indicates that around 70% of men in their 70s will experience

BOX 19.1   Problems affecting arousal in men

Balanitis (inflammation of glans penis)
The glans may appear red and sore, sometimes with whitish streaks or spots or ulcers. Balanitis is usually caused by fungal infection, but may occur after the use of heavily perfumed bath products or in diabetes mellitus. It can be uncomfortable, if not necessarily painful, and can make sexual arousal less pleasant.

Torn frenulum
The frenulum is the ridge of skin that joins the underside of the glans penis to the foreskin in men who have not been circumcised. It can be torn during sexual activity, causing slight bleeding and pain.

Peyronie's disease
Peyronie's disease is the presence of fibrous plaques within the shaft of the penis. These plaques cause bending and angulation of the erect penis, sometimes to the extent that sexual intercourse is impossible. The condition affects men of any age.

The three main symptoms are:
- pain with erections
- a palpable lump in the shaft
- curvature of the penis with erections.

Some men may also develop erectile dysfunction problems.

Although treatment is not always needed, a range of treatments has been developed; none is effective in all cases:

- oral tamoxifen may help prevent formation of fibrous plaques in the early stages
- vitamin E can help ease pain and deformity
- verapamil may help decrease plaque size and pain when injected directly into the plaque
- interferon may also be used in treatment.

Surgery can be an option once the disease has stabilised. This may entail removal of tissue opposite the penile curve, or it may be possible to elongate the plaque by use of a graft. Excision of the fibrous plaque is not advised because it can lead to erectile dysfunction. In some cases, a prosthesis is inserted.

Priapism
A priapism is a prolonged and painful erection that results when blood fails to return as normal from the corpora cavernosa of the penis to the circulation. The condition may occur if disease of the spinal cord or brain disturbs the nervous control of blood flow to and from the penis; drugs used for erectile dysfunction may also contribute.

Priapism is a medical emergency because of the risk of blood clotting. Patients should go without delay to an accident and emergency department.

Paraphimosis
Phimosis refers to a tightness of the foreskin, and a paraphimosis occurs when the foreskin swells around the glans penis. It is a painful condition that can occur after sex if the foreskin is not rolled back into place, and some patients will need to attend the accident and emergency department.

BOX 19.2   Erectile changes that may occur with age[4]

- Longer time to get an erection
- May need more direct stimulation of penis to achieve erection
- Erections may be less firm (but still sufficiently solid for intercourse)
- May be less semen ejaculated
- May feel less need to ejaculate (which may mean more frequent erections)
- May need more rest time between one ejaculation and another
- Older men may make love for longer before needing to ejaculate
- Control over the ejaculation may be far greater
- Ejaculation may be less powerful

difficulty obtaining and maintaining an erection, albeit only occasionally.[8–10]

Treatment

So what can be done to help? Sometimes patients have the idea that a particular remedy is a panacea, Viagra (sildenafil) being a current favourite. However, the choice of treatment for erectile dysfunction will depend upon the cause or causes, hence the need for detailed assessment. It may be necessary to correct misunderstandings and explain the need for an initial medical consultation in addition to outlining the various treatment options.

When erectile dysfunction is psychological in origin, arising from stress and anxiety, patients may respond well to sex counselling. The practice nurse should, therefore, be aware of facilities and resources for this in the practice locality. The system for referral may vary from place to place, so check local protocols and follow established policies.

A wide range of treatments is available for physical problems. Only a selection of treatments is discussed here.

Oral medications are appropriate for some. The celebrated Viagra is one of a group of drugs called phosphodiesterase type-5 inhibitors that work by helping to relax the blood vessels in the penis. Others within this group include Levitra (vardenafil) and Cialis (tadalafil). It may be necessary to explain that the drugs are not aphrodisiacs and do not increase sexual desire. They are not suitable for all men; caution is necessary, especially, for example, in cardiac or renal disease or stroke.[13]

There is an intraurethral medication known as MUSE (Medicated Urethral System for Erection). A special applicator is used to administer the drug into the urethra from where it is absorbed. The principal ingredient is alprostadil, a naturally occurring prostaglandin that helps relax muscles in the penis and allows increased blood flow.[13]

Another option is an injection. Alprostadil (Caverject) is injected straight into the penis, using a needle so fine as to be virtually painless, and produces an erection in almost all men.[1, 2, 13] Of course, the idea of injections does not appeal to all. When teaching a patient how to administer the injection, it is crucial that health professionals convey no sense of distaste or aversion.

These alprostadil preparations and the oral medications for the management of erectile dysfunction are available at NHS expense only in certain circumstances.

Some men seem to find vacuum devices helpful, although for others having to attach mechanical apparatus to the genitals may be off-putting or be seen as inconvenient. Vacuum devices work by drawing blood into the penis. As yet there is little evidence to support their use,[2] so not all health professionals would recommend such devices.

Finally, surgical treatments have been undertaken with varying degrees of success;[4] procedures range from improving the circulation to the penis, to the use of implants and prostheses.

Problems with ejaculation

Problems with ejaculation range from premature ejaculation (one of the most common sexual prob-

TABLE 19.2 Problems affecting ejaculation

Problem	Causes	Treatment
Delayed ejaculation Ejaculation is impaired, and the man finds great difficulty reaching orgasm in spite of stimulation and a desire to do so; relatively uncommon	Causes may be physical (e.g. diabetes mellitus, prostate disease, drug therapy, especially some antidepressants and beta-blockers) or psychological (various stresses and anxieties)	Treatment may entail psychosexual therapy from specialist practitioners (NB: not always available through the NHS)
Retrograde ejaculation The sensation of ejaculation is experienced but initially no seminal fluid is seen; following intercourse, the man may notice his urine appears cloudy. In this condition, the semen enters the bladder rather than being ejected via the urethra	A common cause is prostate or bladder-neck surgery; less common reasons include disruption to the nerve supply in spinal cord injury, diabetes mellitus, multiple sclerosis and some medications, particularly antihypertensives. The sensation of orgasm and ejaculation may also be reduced	Treatment is considered only if fertility is an issue
Anejaculation A relatively uncommon condition where the man does not ejaculate at all	Can result from spinal cord injury, lymph node surgery, diabetes mellitus or multiple sclerosis. Can also be a psychological problem	Treatment is usually only indicated to restore fertility

lems affecting men) to anejaculation (Table 19.2).

Premature ejaculation refers to the condition where a man ejaculates too soon. Defining 'too soon' is, unfortunately, a problem in itself. There is no universally accepted definition, so the most important factor is the perception of the man and his partner. Ultimately, if ejaculation happens sooner than the man and his partner wish, it may be considered 'premature'. However, research on this issue has found that the average time for intercourse is 3 minutes,[3] with many men reporting climax times of less than 1 minute and possibly even before any direct stimulation of the penis (Table 19.3).[4, 5, 14] Given such figures, it is worth considering how realistic the expectations of the man and his partner are.

When considering the causes of premature ejaculation, it is also interesting to note that, while it can occur at any age and in any situation, it is more common among younger men. In turn, this may relate more to the novelty of the sexual experience (e.g. a new partner or different situation) than to the man's age.[13]

Other psychosocial factors that may contribute to premature ejaculation include a partner's illness, family problems, a sense of urgency because

TABLE 19.3 Male climax times (based on questionnaires completed by more than 11,000 men of all ages[14])

Time to orgasm	Proportion of men (%)
50–60 s	21
1–5 min	62
5–10 min	8
10–15 min	2
15–20 min	3
20–30 min	None
30–40 min	3
90+ min	1

of a lack of privacy, fear of failure, unrealistic expectations and a lack of interpersonal skills.[2, 4, 13] Indeed, problems with the relationship can play a big part here, especially if one partner is sexually demanding and there is a lack of communication and trust.

Physiological disorders, such as changes in the prostate gland, arteriosclerosis, diabetes and neurological disorders, may be a component of the problem, but most cases are caused by failure to control the ejaculatory response.

So what can be done to help? Many men can be helped to delay ejaculation using self-help methods, but some may need the expert advice of a sex therapist. The Sexual Dysfunction Association recommends a simple self-help method, which is explained in a factsheet (see Further Information). There are also 'delay' creams and sprays on the market, but there is no evidence to support their use.

ACTIVITY

Consider your work base.

Is there information about male sexual dysfunction available for patients to read and take away?

Is it clear and easy to read?

Where is the information placed?

Could it be better displayed, or positioned in such a way that it can be read or gathered without others observing?

RESPONDING TO A MALE CLIENT WITH A SEXUAL DYSFUNCTION

Given the sensitive nature of sexual dysfunction, it seems almost facile to say that establishing trust and a positive relationship is the key to success. Nevertheless, it is crucial not to underestimate the skills necessary to achieve this; in essence, they are interpersonal skills that demonstrate approachability and a genuine regard for people, and these skills are often more important to patients than a great knowledge of disease processes or particular treatments.

The starting point is self-awareness on the part of the nurse or health professional. We all need to be aware of our own beliefs and value systems, as these will affect the attitudes that we display to others. Being comfortable and confident when talking about sexual issues requires that you reflect on your own understandings, and develop an awareness of how others may feel about such matters.

Getting it wrong can be very damaging for patients and their partners. If you are uncomfortable discussing sexual problems it is much better that you refer patients to others until you have had sufficient opportunity to observe, develop and refine your skills. Ultimately, getting it right is about being yourself: the genuine you. However, the genuine you must hit the right tone when interacting with the patient, adapting your communication style to suit the varying needs of individuals.

Taking the patient seriously when discussing his concerns is also critical. Many will have grown up in an environment in which attitudes were more rigid than they are today, and in consequence may have endured many months of silent misery. They are likely to be feeling very self-conscious when bringing their problems to you. A flippant remark can bring a conversation to an abrupt conclusion – but so too can an 'over-earnest' style of interaction that makes the patient feel like a child or a deviant!

Some men may feel shame because they feel their sexuality is being brought into question. Indeed sexism, ageism and homophobia all interact to create a pervasive mythology about male sexual disorders. Some of these myths were raised earlier in this chapter, but many others may be brought into consultations and need to be clearly corrected without damaging the patient's self-esteem.

ACTIVITY

Think about a situation when you have been asked, or when you might be asked, for advice about male sexual dysfunction.

How did or do you feel about this?

What factors will determine the success of your contribution in such instances?

Much of what the nurse does is concerned with being a resource; one that listens, helps to clarify a particular picture and, as necessary, explains the options available. Many of these options, such as the sex therapist or a GP consultation, are external to the treatment room. However, helping people form realistic expectations of what is available and of what can be achieved is one of the most important parts of health promotion, and a major step in the resolution of problems.

ACTIVITY

Identify the resources available in your area to support men with sexual dysfunction.

Are there local clinics?

Who runs the services?

Discuss with your colleagues what resources are available, and make your own list of them.

CONCLUSION

The issue of male sexual dysfunction is one that presents health professionals with many challenges; not the least of these is the, often acute, embarrassment that may be felt by the patient, which can hinder the communication of problems and concerns. However, through the use of a range of skills and knowledge, practice nurses can, and indeed already do, make a real difference to the promotion of male sexual health. Through a commitment to continue developing knowledge and skills in this area, you can help to prevent much unnecessary suffering, and promote healthy and fulfilling sex lives for your patients.

EVALUATION ACTIVITY

On the basis of what you have learned from this chapter, evaluate the success of any changes you have made to your practice.

LEARNING POINTS

- Sexual difficulties are common, and almost all men will experience one at some point in their lives
- Sexual dysfunction is difficulty engaging in, or inability to engage in, sexual activity, which arises from a physical or psychological disorder or a combination of both. This does not include variations in sexual practice or sexual orientation
- Myth may suggest that men are always ready for and wanting sex, but 'going off it' is not uncommon and occurs for many different reasons
- If you are uncomfortable discussing sexual problems, refer patients to others until you have had sufficient opportunity to observe, develop and refine your skills

---

REFERENCES

1. Clark P. Male order problems. Nursing Times 1997; 93(10): 32–33.
2. Banks I. The Man Manual. Yeovil: Haynes, 2002.
3. Hopcroft K, Moulds A. A Bloke's Diagnose-It-Yourself Guide to Health. Oxford: Oxford University Press, 2000.
4. Bradford N. Men's Health Matters: The Complete A-Z of Male Health. London: Vermilion, 1995.
5. Gebhard P, Johnson A. The Kinsey Data. Philadelphia: Saunders, 1979.
6. Dorey G. Partners' perspective of erectile dysfunction: literature review. Br J Nursing 2001; 10(3): 187–195.
7. Perry A, Schacht M. American Medical Association: Complete Guide to Men's Health. New York: Wiley, 2001.
8. Feldman HA, Goldstein I, Dimitrios GH, Krane RJ, McKinlay JB. Impotence and its medical and psychosocial correlates: results of the Massachusetts Male Aging Study. J Urology 1994; 151: 54–61.

9. Martin C. Factors affecting sexual functioning in 60–79-year old married males. Arch Sex Behav 1981; 10: 399–420.
10. Mulligan T, Moss CR. Sexuality and aging in male veterans: A cross-sectional study of interest, ability and activity. Arch Sex Behav 1991; 20: 17–25.
11. Nadelson CC. Geriatric sex problems: discussion. J Geriatr Psychiatr 1984; 17: 139–148.
12. Wright D. Sex and the elderly. Nurs Mirror 1985; 161(5): 18–19.
13. Sexual Dysfunction Association. Treatment for Impotence. Factsheet. Available at: http://www.sda.uk.net
14. Hite S. The Hite Report on Male Sexuality. New York: Alfred A. Knopf, 1978.

FURTHER INFORMATION

Sexual Dysfunction Association: produces factsheets on erectile dysfunction and related problems. When writing for information send a large SAE. The Sexual Dysfunction Association, Windmill Place Business Centre, 2–4 Windmill Lane, Southall, Middlesex UB2 4NJ. Tel. 08707 743 571; http://www.sda.uk.net

Chapter 20

MALE SEXUAL HEALTH

Prostate cancer: risk, symptoms and investigation

Graham Harris

CHAPTER CONTENTS

LEARNING OBJECTIVES

After reading this chapter you will be able to:

- discuss prostate cancer and identify its clinical features
- explain how the diagnosis is made and how the condition is investigated

---

Prostate cancer is one of the most common cancers to affect men, with almost three times as many men dying from it as do women from cervical cancer.[1,2] In spite of campaigns to raise public awareness and increasing research into new treatments, much remains to be done to ensure prostate cancer receives the attention it deserves.[3–5]

Practice nurses can promote understanding of prostate cancer. Many are actively involved in this area – some are even setting up and running

---

ACTIVITY

Think about prostate cancer.

What do you already know about the condition?

How would you explain it to a patient?

How do the symptoms of prostate cancer differ from other prostate disorders?

---

clinics to support early detection and treatment. An understanding of the disease, treatment options and current developments is important to all practice nurses.

PROSTATE CANCER: EXPLORING THE TERRITORY

Seven men out of 10 are unsure about where the prostate gland is and what it does. Patient education should begin by establishing just how much is understood. Information must be given respectfully and tailored to suit individual needs (Box 20.1). If the patient feels patronised it can end a potentially helpful learning relationship. Once a basic understanding is established, the three main problems that can occur with the prostate can be explained. Prostatitis, benign prostatic hyperplasia (BPH) and prostate cancer all have similar symptoms

Prostatitis is an inflammation of the gland; it causes dysuria and a range of other symptoms, such as urinary frequency and poor or slow urine flow. It can occur at any age but is most common in younger men and may be related to infection with *Chlamydia*.[2]

BPH is the hypertrophy (or overgrowth) of prostatic tissue that is common as men get older.

Symptoms may be similar to those in prostatitis, with difficulty in passing urine and problems such as nocturia, frequency of micturition and poor urinary stream.[6]

In prostate cancer there is again overgrowth of prostatic tissue, but in this case, unlike BPH, the cells that grow can invade healthy tissue and spread to other parts of the body (metastasise).[6] Prostate cancer may not have spread at all when detected. Often it is so slow growing that it is 'latent' and does not cause symptoms or shorten the person's life. There are also aggressive types with a strong likelihood of noticeable symptoms.[7] Initial symptoms may be an obstructed bladder, with problems such as dysuria and poor stream as the enlarging prostate begins to compress the urethra. However, as the condition develops, further less common problems may arise (Box 20.2), including pain on micturition and haematuria, although these are not exclusive to prostate cancer.[6] Some men experience pain in the perineum, describing it as occurring between the scrotum and rectum, or testicular pain – particularly if there is involvement of the nerves serving the perineal area.[8] In others, the first symptoms appear in what seem to be unrelated areas of the body – for example pathological fractures or lumbar pain in cases of bony metastases.

So why do some men develop prostate cancer and, given that many of its symptoms are shared with other non-cancerous disorders, how is it detected? Who is at risk? And why are there no national screening programmes like those for women's cancers – cervical and breast cancer?

BOX 20.1   Information for patients on the prostate gland

The prostate:

- is a small accessory sex gland that lies just below the bladder
- encircles the urethra
- is usually about the size of a walnut
- has two functions at the time of ejaculation – it provides the fluid that nourishes and transports sperm and contributes to the sensations of orgasm

---

ACTIVITY

Think about a person you know with prostate cancer.

What kind of profile does that person present?

How was their cancer detected?

What investigations were performed?

BOX 20.2 Symptoms in prostate cancer at different stages of disease[8]		
Symptoms from an enlarging prostate gland	**Symptoms from the localised spread of prostate cancer**	**Symptoms from metastatic disease**

These symptoms are particularly associated with cancer arising in the transitional zone or inner part of the prostate, which squeezes off the urethra. Of all diagnosed cases, about 30% are in the transitional zone
 	
• The symptoms include:
  – poor urinary flow
  – difficulty in starting (hesitancy)
  – difficulty in finishing cleanly (post-micturition dribbling)
 	
• Secondary to this, the bladder can become irritated as it has to contract harder to push the urine through the narrowed urethra. This may result in:
  – frequency of micturition and nocturia
  – an inappropriately strong urge to urinate
 	
NB: These symptoms are also seen in men with BPH and other disorders
	As the cancer advances, so it may invade surrounding tissues and structures. Specifically localised spread may affect:
	– the bladder and nearby lymph nodes
	– seminal vesicles and the nerves that control erections
	– sensation of the perineal skin
	
	• If the base of the bladder has been invaded, it can cause:
	  – blood in the urine (haematuria)
	  – bladder irritation resulting in urgency and frequency
	
	• Invasion of the seminal vesicles is rare but can result in blood in the ejaculate (haemospermia)
	
	• Local invasion into the nerves can present in a variety of ways – including problems in getting erections, pain in the perineum and pelvic discomfort
	
	NB: These symptoms are also seen in men with other urological disorders
		More than 40% of men diagnosed with prostate cancer still do not present until they have metastatic disease
		
		• Pain resulting from bony metastases, particularly in the pelvis and lumbar spine, is the major symptom, although some men first present with a fracture
		
		• If many vertebrae are involved, spinal compression can occur. This causes weakness in the legs and loss of control of urinary and bowel sphincters
		
		• Other symptoms of distant metastases are sciatica, lymph node enlargement, swelling in the lower limbs
		
		• Widespread metastatic cancer may give rise to more generalised symptoms such as loss of appetite, weight loss and lethargy

RISK FACTORS

There is no easy profile of a typical prostate cancer sufferer because it affects men from all backgrounds and in many different ways. The principal risk factor is age, although the disease is not restricted to those over 70 years old and is becoming more common in those over 50 years old.[9] Half of all cases are in men over 75 years old but this is likely to change.[1, 9] The average age of death from prostate cancer is about 70 years, with an average loss of life expectancy of about 9 years – precious retirement years for which most men have worked all their lives.[8]

Of the other factors, some, such as racial origin, are non-modifiable (Box 20.3). There are others, however, over which men can have some influence, and it is important that these are

BOX 20.3   Risk factors for prostate cancer

- Belonging to an older age group (usually 55+ years)
- Having a close family member who has had prostate cancer
- Having certain racial origins, e.g. it is more common among men of an Afro-Caribbean origin
- Following certain eating patterns, e.g. a high-fat diet
- Low exposure to sunlight
- Working with the element cadmium and working within the nuclear industry

discussed as part of any health promotion programme.[8]

Like breast cancer, cancer of the prostate runs in certain families and a man whose father or brother has had the disease diagnosed before the age of 60 years has a 2–3 times greater risk of developing the disease than a man without an affected relative.[2, 6, 7] In such families, offer all male members regular screening to ensure that any prostate cancer is diagnosed early.

In terms of racial factors, Afro-Caribbean men are at highest risk, seeming to develop an aggressive form of the disease, often at a younger age than caucasians, whereas men of east Asian descent seem much less likely to be affected.[3]

Diet is the first of the modifiable risk factors. Reducing intake of eggs, milk, cheese, butter and red meat may do much to preserve the health of the prostate (and of many other organs). The rationale is that eating a lot of saturated animal fat increases the amount of free radicals in the body, and that these reduce the body's levels of beta-carotene, which reputedly protects against many cancers.[8, 10]

Some practitioners recommend dietary supplements, especially the antioxidants vitamin E, selenium and lycopenes (Table 20.1). Before starting any kind of supplement, however, check the man's medical history and any medications he takes, because interactions may occur. Those wary of dietary supplements may prefer to eat food sources.

Prostate cancer is more common in countries at higher latitudes, with Norway and Sweden having the highest death rates.[8] As exposure to sunlight helps the body to produce vitamin D, this suggests that low vitamin D could be another risk factor.

Men who work in the nuclear industry have a higher incidence of prostate cancer but the exact cause of this relationship is unknown.[8] Cadmium, a mineral of no known function in the body, has also been associated with the disease, as have high levels of testosterone and a testosterone–oestrogen imbalance.[9, 10]

DETECTION AND INVESTIGATION

Well-established examinations and investigations are used to detect prostate cancer. Encouraging

TABLE 20.1   Specific dietary intakes suggested for prostate health

Supplement/ food stuffs	Recommended daily intake	Notes
Vitamin E	400 IU	Rarely (if ever) deficient in a balanced diet.[10] Functions as an antioxidant in cell membranes – protecting unsaturated fatty acids from oxidative damage
Selenium	200 µg	A mineral that acts as an antioxidant. Sources include fish, kidney beans, Brazil nuts, liver, lentils, pork, veal
Lycopenes	15 mg	Red pigment found in tomato skins, pink grapefruit and palm oil. An antioxidant

men to present promptly is critical, because in about 40% of cases the disease has spread at the time of diagnosis. This may be local (into the bladder and surrounding structures) or to areas such as the bones of the pelvis and lumbar spine.[8, 11]

History

A detailed history is necessary, with careful consideration of symptoms. Some practitioners advocate self-administered symptom questionnaires (Box 20.4). These are a means of establishing the severity of problems and may help patients to identify issues they might otherwise not report. Remember, however, that a symptom questionnaire is not a diagnostic tool – only a means to gain an understanding of how the person perceives their experiences.

The impact of symptoms on the individual, his partner and family is often considerable so it is important to acknowledge this. Disturbed nights, for example, can affect all members of the household. Broken sleep and discomfort from symptoms such as urgency and frequency can take a huge toll on relationships – with strained emotions and frayed nerves.

Examination

A digital rectal examination (DRE) is usually the first investigation to follow history taking.[11–13] It provides invaluable information but is a skilled procedure and should only be undertaken after appropriate training. Men often find the prospect of the DRE quite alarming, and to avoid embarrassment it must be explained and performed with sensitivity. Some may be reassured by the fact that, while the examination may be disagreeable, with some discomfort, it is over very quickly – usually taking no more than a couple of minutes.

The man should be asked to lie in the left lateral position with his knees brought up towards his chest – in the 'fetal position'. A gloved, lubricated index finger is then inserted via the anal sphincter – so the posterior part of the prostate can be palpated through the rectal wall. Advise the patient to breathe deeply and evenly, as this may help him to relax.

The aim of the DRE is to feel the size, shape and texture of the gland. Prostatic tumours often arise on the periphery, which is why it is possible for them to be detected in this way, and a nodule or hard, indurated area, or pronounced asymmetry may be felt. However, it is unlikely that small tumours will be palpated using this procedure so it must be emphasised that it is not a fail-safe test.

PROSTATE SPECIFIC ANTIGEN TEST

The next investigation to consider is the blood test known as the PSA – the prostate specific antigen test. PSA is a protein secreted exclusively by the epithelial cells of the prostate and its serum concentration is raised in men with prostatic diseases.[13–17] A very high 'total PSA' result is suggestive of advanced prostate cancer. A 'raised' PSA level is considered to be above 4 ng/ml, exact interpretation depending on factors such as the patient's age and whether they have undergone recent urological investigations (Box 20.5).[15]

The PSA test is controversial and there is debate about whether it should be provided for all men over 50 years old as part of a screening programme. For more on this aspect see Chapter 21. There is also an issue about the nature of the test. PSA can exist in different forms in the blood – it can be 'complexed' (bound to other proteins), or exist alone as 'free PSA'.[7] Generally, the tests used measure total PSA. Yet the relative proportions of free and complexed PSA are believed to differ in cancer and in other prostate diseases, and it is thought that men with prostate cancer will have less free PSA and more of the complexed variety.[11] In consequence, some have been lobbying for use of the cPSA test, which takes this into account.

BOX 20.4   The International Prostate Symptom Scoring Chart, developed by WHO[14]

Self Assessment

The International Prostate Symptom Score is a questionnaire – containing seven questions about the symptoms you may be experiencing. Select the response for each question that most closely corresponds to your experiences.

To mark your response, tick in the column that best describes your symptom or circle the score. After you answer these seven questions, your score will be calculated immediately, and you will be given a brief interpretation of the score. Please feel free to ask any questions that you have about the score results.

INTERNATIONAL PROSTATE SYMPTOM SCORE
Tick or circle only once in each category

Questions to be answered regarding your BPH condition	Not at all	Less than 1 time in 5	Less than half the time	About half the time	More than half the time	Almost always	Point value
Over the past month, how often have you had a sensation of not emptying your bladder completely after you finished urinating?	0	1	2	3	4	5	
Over the past month, how often have you had to urinate again less than 2 hours after you finished urinating?	0	1	2	3	4	5	
Over the past month, how often have you stopped and started again several times when you urinated?	0	1	2	3	4	5	
Over the past month, how often have you found it difficult to postpone urination?	0	1	2	3	4	5	
Over the past month, how often have you had a weak urinary stream?	0	1	2	3	4	5	
Over the past month, how often have you had to push or strain to begin urination?	0	1	2	3	4	5	
Over the past month, how many times did you most typically get up to urinate from the time you went to bed at night until the time you got up in the morning? (Tick in the column which best represents the number of times you awake each night, on average)	0 times	1 times	2 times	3 times	4 times	5 times	
							Score

What your score means

0–7 points   Symptoms are considered mild
8–19 points   Symptoms are considered moderate
20–35 points   Symptoms are considered severe

This index is a guide for determining the severity of your symptoms. It does NOT diagnose a specific condition or disease

---

BOX 20.5   Key messages about the PSA test[15]

1. Prostate specific antigen (PSA) is a tumour marker – sometimes helpful as a screening tool in the detection of prostate cancer, for the staging of cancer and for measuring response to treatment

2. Serum values of PSA are not generally affected by digital rectal examination (DRE) but can be affected by other urological tests and prostate biopsy

3. Other, non-malignant conditions can elevate PSA levels including prostatitis and BPH

4. The normal range of PSA is considered to be between 0 and 4 ng/ml. However, some practitioners consider age ranges too:

Age range (years)	PSA (ng)
40–49	2.5
50–59	3.5
60–69	4.5
70–79	6.5

5. In large-scale screening it has been found that 5–10% of a population will have an abnormal PSA, and about one in five patients with a PSA of 4.0–10 ng/ml will have prostate cancer, whereas about 60% of patients with a PSA > 10 ng/ml will have cancer

6. A PSA test should be performed in combination with a DRE because it is suggested that PSA alone will miss about 20% of tumours

---

If the PSA is raised and especially if the DRE is also abnormal, further investigations will be needed – usually a prostate biopsy. The aim is to confirm the presence of cancer and then to grade it on the Gleason scale (discussed in Chapter 21). There are two components to the procedure: transrectal ultrasonography (TRUS) and the biopsies themselves.

Prophylactic antibiotics may be given before the procedure as well as a local anaesthetic. Biopsy is considered to be uncomfortable but rarely requires general anaesthetic. The patient is instructed to adopt the same position as for a DRE. When he is comfortable, a lubricated ultrasound probe can be gently introduced into the rectum.

The high-frequency sound waves emitted from the probe bounce off the surrounding structures back to the probe. These echoes can then be used to produce an image of the prostate on a computer screen. Again, irregularity in the shape or consistency or defects in the capsule are noted. The biopsy needle is inserted through a port in the probe and then advanced into the prostate. Up to 12 cores of tissue will be removed from all areas of the gland and any suspicious area will be targeted.

LEARNING POINTS

- Prostatitis, benign prostatic hyperplasia (BPH), and prostate cancer all have similar symptoms
- In cancer the cells that make up the overgrowth of prostatic tissue can invade healthy tissue and spread
- Often the cancer is so slow growing that it does not cause symptoms or shorten the person's life
- The principal risk factor for prostate cancer is age
- Cancer of the prostate runs in certain families
- Digital rectal examination (DRE) is usually the first investigation to follow history taking

---
EVALUATION ACTIVITY

Reflect critically on the care of men with prostate cancer. In particular consider the care they receive when undergoing investigations.

Identify the strengths in clinical care and areas where you wish to develop your practice

---

After the biopsy procedure, oral antibiotics will be continued and patients will need to be advised that blood might be visible in urine or faeces for a few days and may be seen in the semen for several weeks. Even with the antibiotics, there is a risk of urinary tract infection so advice should be given in respect of reporting symptoms such as cloudy or smelly urine, burning and frequency of voiding or generally feeling unwell with pyrexia.

The biopsied tissue enables the likely extent and nature of the cancer to be established. Along with the PSA reading, and how far, if at all, the cancer has spread outside the prostate, it will act as a guide to treatment options.

REFERENCES

1. Cancer Research UK. Prostate Cancer Statistics 2002. London: Cancer Research UK, 2002.
2. Bradford N. Men's Health Matters: The Complete A–Z of Male Health. London: Vermilion, 1995.
3. The Prostate Cancer Charity: http://www.prostate-cancer.org.uk
4. Derbyshire D. Surgeons Pioneer New Treatment For Prostate Cancers. Daily Telegraph, 6 November 2004, p. 8.
5. Derbyshire D. New Way to Beat Prostate Cancer. Daily Telegraph, 6 November 2004, p. 4.
6. Kirk D. Understanding Prostate Disorders. Poole: Family Doctor Publications, 2004.
7. NHS Prostate Cancer Risk Management Statistics: http://www.cancerscreening.nhs.uk/prostate/statistics.html
8. The Prostate Cancer Research Organisation: http://www.prostate-research.org.uk
9. Banks I. The Man Manual. Yeovil: Haynes, 2002.
10. Bender DA. Oxford Dictionary of Food & Nutrition. Oxford: OUP, 2005.
11. The Orchid Cancer Appeal. Prostate Cancer: Important Messages for Men: http://www.orchid-cancer.org.uk
12. Mead M. Aids to General Practice, 2nd edn. Edinburgh: Churchill Livingstone, 1990.
13. Marshall F. Your Man's Health. London: Sheldon Press, 2002.
14. International Prostate Symptom Score (IPSS): http://www.patient.co.uk/showdoc/23069171
15. Prostate Cancer: A Patient's Guide: http://www.medic8.com/healthguide/articles/prostateca.html
16. Timby BK. Fundamental Nursing Skills and Concepts, 8th edn. Philadelphia: Lippincott, Williams & Wilkins, 2005.
17. Catalona W, Smith D, Ratcliff T, Dodds K, Coplen J, Yuan J, Petros J, Andriole G. Measurement of prostate-specific-antigen in serum as a screening test for prostate cancer. N Engl J Med 1991; 324(17): 1156–1161.

FURTHER INFORMATION

Kirk D. Understanding Prostate Disorders. Poole: Family Doctor Publications, 2004.

NHS Website: http://www.cancerscreening.nhs.uk/prostate/index.html

The Prostate Cancer Charity: e-mail: info@prostate-cancer.org.uk; helpline 0845 300 8383; http://www.prostate-cancer.org.uk

Chapter 21

MALE SEXUAL HEALTH

Prostate cancer: grading and staging, screening and treatment

Graham Harris

LEARNING OBJECTIVES

After reading this chapter you will be able to:

- explain the management of prostate cancer, including current treatment strategies
- discuss the issues around screening for prostate cancer
- referring also to Chapter 20, develop (or review the contents of) a health education programme to promote understanding of prostate cancer and its treatment

Prostate cancer is a significant men's health issue, and a condition that presents health professionals with many challenges. In order to establish the best treatment for an individual patient the cancer must first be detected and then assessed.

GRADING AND STAGING PROSTATE CANCER

Grading a prostate cancer can help indicate how aggressive the cancer is. The Gleason grading system, named after the pathologist who devised it, requires calculation of the Gleason Score. First, each tissue sample is graded on a scale from 1 to 5, according to the type of cells seen. Scores of 1 or 2 indicate a slow-growing cancer, sometimes

151

termed 'well-differentiated' as, under the microscope, the cells are still easily identified as prostatic in origin. A score of 5, on the other hand, indicates an aggressive cancer as the highly malignant cells are 'poorly differentiated' and would be difficult to identify as coming from the prostate.

When all tissue specimens have been graded, the grades of the two highest-graded specimens are added together. The total score can thus range from 2 to 10. A Gleason Score of 6 or 7 is quite common and carries a relatively reasonable prognosis, whereas a score of 8 or over indicates a highly malignant and rapidly growing cancer (Table 21.1).[1]

The cancer can also be classified according to how far it has spread – its 'stage' – and the tumour–nodes–metastasis (TNM) staging system is commonly used. An assessment is made of how far the cancer has spread in and around the prostate (Table 21.2), whether it has spread to the nearby lymph nodes and then whether it has spread to the distant lymph nodes and bones. Knowing the stage of the cancer helps to identify the most appropriate course of action.

BONE AND BODY SCANNING

Bone scans may be necessary if the cancer is thought to have spread outside the prostate. MRI (magnetic resonance imaging) and CT (computerised tomography) scans may similarly help to assess the extent of the cancer and whether there is local spread. They can also check whether secondary tumours have formed in other regions.

PROSTATE CANCER: TO SCREEN OR NOT TO SCREEN?

You might wonder why there is no routine screening for prostate cancer. It may seem that a simple blood test to check for a raised level of prostate specific antigen (PSA) could be part of

TABLE 21.1 Prostate cancer survival rates associated with the Gleason Score

Gleason Score	Survival rate
7 or below	87% will survive over 10 years
8 or above	Only 26% survive over 10 years

TABLE 21.2 Simplified staging classification for tumours of the prostate gland

Stage	Interpretation
T1	Non-palpable tumour
T2	Nodule
T3	Extracapsular (outside the prostate gland)

annual health monitoring for all men over 50 years of age.[2] However, the issue is not straightforward and there are advantages and disadvantages to consider (Box 21.1).

Although a 'normal' PSA test result might seem reassuring, the test can miss cancer and give false reassurance. It can also give an abnormal result when there are problems other than cancer, causing much anxiety and possibly unnecessary

BOX 21.1 Consequences of a national programme to screen for raised levels of prostate specific antigen (PSA)[3]

If a national programme of PSA testing were to be introduced:

- some men would be diagnosed with cancer at an early stage when treatment would help
- some men with cancer would be missed
- some men without cancer would be encouraged to undergo unnecessary investigations
- some men with slow-growing cancers would be given treatment that they probably did not need

tests when no cancer is present. The stance of Cancer Research UK on the issue – that there is no evidence that a national screening programme would reduce the number of deaths from prostate cancer – is also adopted within the NHS website.[3, 4]

TREATMENTS

A wide range of treatments is available for men with prostate cancer so it is important that nurses are aware of the options. Patients may want to discuss them, and some will have questions and anxieties raised by reading newspapers or information they have found on the internet.

Treatment for cancers contained within the prostate

When the cancer has not spread beyond the prostate gland, treatment options range from 'active surveillance' to radical prostatectomy, radiotherapy and cryotherapy. These options are discussed in turn below, and the decision depends on several factors, including the patient's choice. The quality of information given, how advanced the cancer is (grade and stage), and the patient's general health will all influence this decision. The goal is for all parties – the patient, his family and the professionals involved – to feel happy with the chosen treatment.

Active surveillance

The term 'active surveillance' has replaced 'watchful waiting', which some considered implied 'doing nothing' when this is not so. Active surveillance entails regular check-ups and monitoring, including repeat PSA tests, and may be appropriate for those whose life expectancy is limited by extreme age or another life-shortening medical condition. For some individuals, in whom the chance of a small tumour causing problems before the end of life is relatively small, it is a way of promoting maximum quality of life. The risk can also be balanced against possible side-effects from other treatments.

If the active surveillance option is chosen, the patient must be convinced it is right for him. There also needs to be good communication. If an individual experiences anxiety that affects his sleep or ability to enjoy everyday activities, then his quality of life will suffer and the team caring for him will need to know, because it may be appropriate to offer alternative treatments.

Radical prostatectomy

Radical prostatectomy entails surgical removal of the entire prostate along with the seminal vesicles and the nearest lymph glands. The procedure is intended to be curative and is therefore offered only to men whose cancer is confined to the prostate gland.[2] The operation can be performed using one of three approaches:

- retropubically – the option most widely used[3]
- via the perineum
- laparoscopically.

Samples from the lymph nodes nearest to the prostate are taken at the time of the surgery to check whether or not cancer has spread to these sites.

A nerve-sparing technique is used to minimise disturbance to the 'cavernous' nerves that are situated in bundles at each side of the prostate and are important for achieving an erection. Although every effort is made to protect this function, erectile dysfunction follows surgery in 30–50% of patients and some men will require

---

ACTIVITY

Think of a person you know with prostate cancer.

What treatments were they offered?

What were the side-effects of the treatments?

How would you describe the various treatments that can be given?

other treatments to help overcome this.[2, 3, 5, 6] The other disadvantage of radical prostatectomy is that many patients experience a temporary loss of continence; sometimes this lasts for months post-operatively and 2–5% of patients will have a long-term problem.[3, 6]

After surgery, the PSA level is monitored. If the operation has been successful, PSA should remain almost undetectable at less than 0.1 ng/ml. Sadly, in almost one-third of men it is found that the cancer has spread outside the prostate, so a course of radiotherapy or drugs may also be required. That said, about 80% of men are alive 10 years after surgery, and 60% at 15 years.[6–8]

Radiotherapy

Radiotherapy can be an alternative and an adjunct to radical prostatectomy. Used alone, radiotherapy has achieved similar survival rates to radical prostatectomy and it is therefore considered app-ropriate for men whose cancer is confined to the prostate, especially if the tumour is of a high Gleason grade.[3] However, it is also suitable for men whose general health precludes major surgery.

Patients may be offered external-beam radio-therapy or brachytherapy. The most commonly used is external-beam radiotherapy, which is usually given over a 6-week period as an out-patient procedure. The treatment requires short sessions 5 days a week, with weekends off as 'rest periods', although some patients need longer breaks to recuperate.

Hormone treatment (explained later) for 3 months before the radiotherapy improves long-term survival and is widely used.[3, 5, 7] It is believed to shrink the prostate so that the cancer cells are concentrated in a smaller area and more likely to be 'hit' by the radiation.

The main side-effects of radiotherapy relate to urinary problems and erectile dysfunction. Usually these effects are mild but if problems are severe, a rest from radiotherapy will often settle them.

Erectile dysfunction occurs in fewer than one-third of patients; it is of gradual rather than sudden onset, and can be overcome with treat-ment. Irritation or discomfort around the rectum, sometimes accompanied by diarrhoea and bleed-ing, is a mostly temporary side-effect that lasts only a few weeks.[3]

Brachytherapy entails insertion into the prostate of 60–100 radioactive seeds, so that radiation is emitted from inside the prostate rather than from an external source. The seeds are left in place and gradually lose their radioactivity over a period of months. Localisation of the radiation makes side-effects such as incontinence less common, but the treatment is suitable only for small tumours so its use is limited.[3, 5]

Cryotherapy

Cryotherapy is administered by means of a probe or specially designed needles that are inserted into the prostate to freeze the cancerous cells and thereby cause cell death. The principal risk associated with this treatment is damage to the urethra or rectum during the freezing process. Further, many patients experience bladder irri-tation with urgency and frequency, although this settles with time. This treatment is of particular interest because it can be used with men whose cancer returns after a course of radiotherapy.[5]

Treatment in locally advanced prostate cancer

When prostate cancer has spread outside the prostate, but not to nearby lymph nodes or more distant locations, it is described as being 'locally advanced'. There is controversy about the best method of treatment; the options include active surveillance, hormone therapy, intermittent hor-mone therapy, hormone therapy followed by radical prostatectomy and, finally, hormone therapy followed by radiotherapy.[1]

Active surveillance

Active surveillance has different connotations when the cancer is more advanced, and therefore likely to become life-threatening more quickly than a low-grade cancer confined to the prostate. Hence, this option may be more suited to those patients with a poor life expectancy.

Hormone therapy

Hormone therapy has a long history in the treatment of prostate cancer. The underlying principle is that testosterone, the male hormone produced in the testes, stimulates prostate cancer growth. The aim is to reduce the effect of testosterone by stopping or 'switching off' its production and/or reducing its effects on the cancer. Ultimately, this will reduce tumour size and delay progression to metastatic or life-threatening stages.[2, 3, 5] Clearly, it is critical that the patient understands that the therapy is not a cure.

Hormone therapy is administered in one of two ways:

- as implants injected into the fat below the skin on the abdomen at monthly or 3-monthly intervals
- daily in tablet form.

The injected drugs, known as luteinising hormone-releasing hormone analogues (LHRH analogues), work by stopping the production of testosterone. As a consequence, men receiving them are likely to experience a loss in sex drive and will probably be unable to achieve erection. However, these effects are gradually reversed once the drug is stopped. The drugs used include goserelin (Zoladex), leuprorelin (Prostap SR) and triptorelin (Decapeptyl).[5]

The hormone tablets are usually anti-androgens and generally work by preventing the action of testosterone on the tumour, without reducing circulating testosterone levels.[1] As a result, they have less effect on libido and erections than the implants, although they may cause stomach upsets and diarrhoea. Rarely, they can adversely affect liver function, so regular blood tests are necessary for monitoring. The drugs used include flutamide (Drogenil) and nilutamide (Anandrone).[5]

A drug often used that works in a slightly different way is cyproterone acetate. Taken in tablet form it not only prevents the action of testosterone but also, because it is similar to a type of female hormone, reduces blood testosterone levels.

Stilboesterol and other female oestrogen hormones were at one time used often to treat prostate cancer. However, their side-effects can include breast-tissue enlargement and cardiac problems so their use has diminished as new hormone medications have developed.[6]

Intermittent hormone therapy

In intermittent hormone therapy, a hormone (an LHRH analogue) is given for a period to shrink the tumour; the treatment is then stopped and re-started when the cancer starts to grow back. The rationale here is that if hormones are given constantly, the cancer will eventually become resistant to them – a situation called 'hormone escape'.

The decision about when to start and stop the LHRH is usually based on PSA levels. This treatment is well evaluated by patients but research continues to establish its comparative merits.[3]

Hormone therapy followed by radical prostatectomy

Evaluation of this treatment continues, although currently many urologists and oncologists do not feel that it is a justifiable option and, therefore, few will recommend its use.[3]

Hormone therapy followed by radiotherapy

According to the Prostate Cancer Research Organisation, results from several large studies show that 3 months of hormone therapy given before starting radiotherapy increases the latter's efficacy, with an increased survival in men at 3 years' follow-up.[3] The studies are ongoing, but in the light of the positive interim results this treatment plan is now used.

Treatment in metastatic disease

It is important that patients with metastatic cancer understand that their cancer has spread to the lymph nodes and to distant sites, such as the bones. They may also need to be made aware that their outlook is relatively poor: about 70% of such patients will have died from their cancer within 5 years.[3, 5]

Nevertheless, treatment options that can delay death for several years include:

- orchidectomy
- hormone therapies (considered by some as the most effective treatment)[1]
- bisphosphonates.

Orchidectomy

Orchidectomy, the surgical removal of the testes, has been shown to be effective; most patients will respond, with the progress of their cancer slowing markedly for about 18 months. However, as the body is rendered unable to produce testosterone, there is also loss of libido and the ability to attain an erection.[1–3, 5]

Hormone therapy

A similar range of drugs is used for the hormone therapy in metastatic disease as already discussed. However, there is also maximal androgen blockade to consider. This combines the use of LHRH analogues with long-term anti-androgens.[5] Some professionals believe this approach is particularly appropriate for younger, relatively fit men.

Bisphosphonates

Bisphosphonates are a group of drugs used to treat osteoporosis, particularly in older women. Their use in men with bony metastases from prostate cancer is still undergoing research, but it already seems that they may have a place in reducing bone pain and in preventing fractures. The most commonly used bisphosphonates are zoledronic acid and clodronate.[3, 5]

Palliative care

Having considered some of the treatments used in metastatic disease, it is appropriate to make a brief mention of the care of patients entering the last stages of their illness. A palliative care team can offer a wide range of support, including referral for various therapies. In bone pain arising from a metastasis, for example, a short course of radiotherapy may be particularly helpful, giving long-term relief.

Significantly, it is often at this point of the illness that patients and their families explore alternative medicines and therapies, and this is an issue they may wish to discuss with nurses. Indeed, the role of the practice nurse in palliative care is substantial, as so many patients and their families will perceive the practice nurse as their 'family nurse'; if a good relationship is established, the nurse will be called upon repeatedly for advice, counselling and sometimes practical help.

MANAGEMENT ISSUES

Throughout this chapter, various aspects of the care and management of men with prostate cancer have been identified. The implications for practice nurses are extensive; developments in this field are rapid and, perhaps more than ever before, nurses are regularly sought out for their knowledge and skilled counsel. From health promotion to support with end-of-life issues, the demands are considerable.

The questions to which nurses are required to respond are varied and often complex. For example, some men may have read about a 'revolutionary' technique in prostate cancer that uses high-intensity focused ultrasound (HIFU), a non-invasive, reputedly painless procedure delivered on a day-case basis.[8, 9] In this case the treatment is only just about to start trials in the UK, so little can be added to what patients may have read for themselves.

ACTIVITY

Consider your work base.

Is there information about prostate cancer available for patients to read and take away?

Is it clear and easy to read?

Where is the information placed?

Could it be better displayed?

Are there information resources for families and carers?

Consider developing, with your colleagues, a resource pack to include information on the different types of treatment and local support groups and services available.

Other more practical considerations may include discussing postoperative recovery after radical prostatectomy. Hospitals may give advice sheets or other forms of patient education; however, it is often the practice nurse who is called upon to reinforce facts, and advise, for example, on the need for more rest as healing takes place, or to avoid heavy lifting in the first 6 weeks to prevent strain on the abdominal wound. Similar support may be required when patients start radiotherapy or other treatments.

Psychological and psychosocial aspects of care sometimes seem low on the agenda in the face of so many new technologies and treatment regimens. Yet, as most nurses will verify, it is often the emotional issues that burden the patient and his partner or family, not only in the early stages of illness or during waits for results from investigations, but sometimes as treatment begins or at later stages.

Never forget how terrifying the word cancer can be. A diagnosis of prostate cancer can lead to sleep disturbance, with the patient chewing over all manner of anxieties, from who will help with the gardening to whether he may have to give up sharing the warmth and comfort of a double bed because of incontinence. Such issues are no mere trifles; they are real, sometimes painful and often very poignant.

A nurse's considered words can be a real help once the patient (or his partner/family/carer) has been given the opportunity to offload concerns and ask their burning questions. Sensitive, well informed responses can really help them to make sense of their situation when a diagnosis of prostate cancer has been made: to discard false hope and destructive hopelessness, and face the future.

CONCLUSION

Practice nurses can, and indeed already do, make a substantial contribution to the management of prostate cancer in primary care. This may include

---

LEARNING POINTS

- Prostate cancer can be graded using the Gleason system: the higher the score (1–10), the more aggressive the cancer. It can also be classified according to degree of spread using the tumour–nodes–metastasis (TNM) system
- Routine screening using the PSA test is a controversial issue. However, leading authorities assert there is no evidence that a national screening programme would reduce the number of related deaths
- Treatments depend on the stage and classification of the disease and on patient choice. They range from active surveillance through surgery and radiotherapy to various drugs and hormone treatments
- Practice nurses have a significant role in prevention and management; from health education and promotion to support and monitoring, there are many challenges that require knowledge, positive and sensitive attitudes and a wide skills base

health promotion advice, assessment and detection of problems, support during investigations and diagnosis, care and management while the patient undergoes treatment, right through to end-of-life care. Only by continuing to raise awareness of prostate cancer, with a genuine commitment to the value of care management for our patients, can we ensure the highest quality of care.

> ## EVALUATION ACTIVITY
>
> In light of what you have learnt in this chapter, update your practice protocol for the monitoring of male patients with prostate cancer.
>
> Reflect critically on your own knowledge and clinical practice, and identify your strengths and areas for development.

REFERENCES

1. Prostate Cancer – A Patient's Guide. http://www.medic8.com/healthguide/articles/prostateca.html
2. Bradford N. Men's Health Matters – The Complete A–Z of Male Health. London: Vermilion, 1995.
3. The Prostate Cancer Research Organisation. http://www.prostate-research.org.uk
4. NHS Prostate Cancer Risk Management Statistics. http://www.cancerscreening.nhs.uk/prostate/statistics.html
5. Kirk D. Understanding Prostate Disorders. Poole: Family Doctor Publications, 2004.
6. Banks I. The Man Manual. Yeovil: Haynes, 2002.
7. Cancer Research UK. Prostate Cancer Statistics 2002. London: Cancer Research UK, 2002.
8. Derbyshire D. Surgeons pioneer new treatment for prostate cancers. The Daily Telegraph, 6 November 2004, p. 8.
9. Derbyshire D. New way to beat prostate cancer. The Daily Telegraph, 6 November 2004, p. 4.

FURTHER INFORMATION

NHS Website: http://www.cancerscreening.nhs.uk/prostate/key-prostate.html

The Prostate Cancer Charity, 3 Angel Walk, Hammersmith, London W6 9HX; Tel. 020 8222 7622; helpline 0845 300 8383; e-mail: info@prostate-cancer.org.uk; http://www.prostate-cancer.org.uk

Health promotion: cardiovascular disease

Chapter 22

CARDIOVASCULAR DISEASE
Coronary heart disease

Sarah Kraszewski

LEARNING OBJECTIVES

After reading this chapter you will be able to:

- demonstrate awareness of the scale of CHD in the UK
- identify national initiatives to improve CHD outcomes
- outline the anatomy and physiology of the heart
- describe the risk factors for CHD

The chapters in this section look at the scale of coronary heart disease (CHD) as a health issue in the UK, review the anatomy and physiology of the heart and consider CHD risk factors.

Heart and circulatory disease is the UK's leading killer.[1] CHD is common, often preventable and largely fatal.[2] Statistics from the British Heart Foundation (BHF) record that, in 2002, 125,000 women died from heart and circulatory disease, almost 2.7 million people had CHD and 662,000 had heart failure. Physical inactivity, smoking and diabetes are major risk factors for CHD (Box 22.1), and in the UK the population exhibits low rates of physical activity and a rising prevalence of obesity.[1] The number of revascularisations performed has increased by one-third since 1999.[1] However, the number of deaths fell from 121,000 in 2001 to 117,500 in 2002[1] and heart disease, for many, is avoidable through simple measures

---

BOX 22.1 Risk factors for CHD

The Framingham Study began in the 1940s, with the aim of generating information on the early detection and prevention of CHD. This longitudinal study has provided valuable information about the relationship between different risk factors for CHD.[12]

CHD risk factors are listed below. Smoking, hypertension and hyperlipidaemia are independent and modifiable risk factors, and the evidence suggests a causal relationship with CHD.[12]

Lifestyle
- Tobacco smoking
- Diet high in saturated fat and calories, high in sugar, low in fruit and vegetables
- Physical inactivity
- Stress
- Excess alcohol
- Obesity

Biochemical or physiological
- Raised blood pressure
- Raised plasma cholesterol
- Low plasma HDL cholesterol
- Raised plasma triglycerides
- Diabetes mellitus
- Thrombogenic factors

Personal
- Age (risk increases above 30 years)
- Sex (up to 60 years, risk is higher in men)
- Family history of CHD (in first-degree relatives)
- Personal history

Family history
Family history is significant if a first CHD event occurred in a first-degree male relative before the age of 55 years, or in a first-degree female relative before the age of 65 years.[14]

Families may exhibit clusters of risk factors, both genetic and environmental. A positive family history facilitates early identification of high-risk individuals.

Ethnic origin may also be a risk factor. South Asians living in the UK have a higher than average death rate from CHD.[15]

Age and sex
CHD incidence increases after the age of 30 years in both sexes. Up to 60 years of age, CHD is more common in men than women, probably because of the protective effect of circulating oestrogen in the premenopausal years. In women over 60 the incidence accelerates until prevalence is fairly equal from the age of 70.[12]

The same risk factors affect men and women, but their relative weightings have important implications for prevention in women.

There is also evidence of under-diagnosis of CHD in women compared with men, and of inequalities in treatment. This may be attributable to the later presentation of CHD in women, and the fact that women more often present with angina than with myocardial infarction.[13]

Stress
Stress is difficult to define – stress for one person may be a challenge to another. However, adverse effects of stress in relation to CHD risk include effects on blood pressure, heart rate, lipids and coagulation mechanisms.[16] Emerging evidence suggests a link between working conditions and CHD: people in jobs where there is poor variety, high intensity and little locus of control are thought to be at higher risk.[13]

Diabetes
Types 1 and 2 diabetes increase CHD risk, and CHD is the leading cause of death in people with diabetes.[12] Approaches to risk reduction for this patient group must be multifaceted and intense.

taken to improve lifestyles. The practice nurse can play a major part in facilitating patients' efforts to change risky behaviours.

ACTIVITY

Reflect upon your role in health promotion.

How do you approach patients to discuss risk factors and healthy living?

ANATOMY AND PHYSIOLOGY OF THE HEART

The heart is a pump of incredible strength and endurance. It is located in the mediastinum, resting superiorly on the diaphragm, anterior to the vertebral column and posterior to the sternum.[3] Enclosing the heart is the pericardium, a double-walled sac comprising an outer fibrous layer and an inner serous layer.

The heart wall has three layers: the outer epicardium, the central myocardium and the inner endocardium. The epicardium is the visceral layer of the serous pericardium. The myocardium forms the bulk of the heart and consists of contractile cardiac muscle.

Cardiac muscle is made up of individual cells, which are electrically connected. Depolarisation of the cells causes contraction and the electrical connections allow the wave of contraction to move across the myocardium.[4]

The myocardium depends upon aerobic respiration and is impaired by oxygen deficiency. The endocardium consists of endothelial tissue, and lines the inside of the heart, covering the valves and the joining vessels, to ensure a smooth flow of blood.[3]

Chambers and vessels

The heart has four chambers: two superior atria and two inferior ventricles. The longitudinal dividing structure is known as the septum.

The left and right atria are the smaller, low-pressure receiving chambers; the thicker walled ventricles pump blood out into the pulmonary and systemic circulations. Four valves ensure that circulation is a one-way system.[3]

The right atrium receives deoxygenated blood returning from the body at low pressure, from the inferior and superior vena cava and the coronary sinus. This blood moves via the tricuspid valve from the right atrium to the right ventricle, from where it is pumped through the pulmonary valve to the pulmonary arteries. These carry blood to the lungs, and are the only arteries in the body to carry deoxygenated blood.

The blood is oxygenated as it passes through the lungs, gas exchange occurring through the alveoli, and the oxygenated blood returns to the left atrium via the pulmonary veins, which are the only veins in the body to carry oxygenated blood. From the left atrium the blood flows via the mitral (bicuspid) valve into the left ventricle, from where it is propelled through the aortic valve into the aorta and so into the high-pressure systemic circulation.

The heart's contractions are controlled by a specialised group of pacemaker cells located in the sino-atrial node. From this node a rhythmic depolarisation of the myocardial cells spreads over the atria, causing atrial contraction that moves blood into the ventricles.

The electrical conduction then passes via the atrioventricular node to the bundle of His. This band of atypical cardiac muscle fibres divides at the upper end of the interventricular septum into left and right bundle branches and propagates the atrial contraction rhythm to the ventricles, via the Purkinje fibres, leading to ventricular contraction.

Contraction of the heart, especially that of the ventricles, is known as systole and the relaxation period as diastole.[4]

To function effectively, the heart needs a blood supply of its own. The myocardium is supplied via the left and right coronary arteries, which are the first branches of the aorta.

The systemic circulation consists of arteries, capillaries and veins. The arteries are muscular tubes designed to carry blood under pressure.

The thinner walled veins carry blood back to the heart at lower pressure; they rely on muscular movement (e.g. of the calf muscle in the case of lower-leg veins) to move the blood along them, and have valves that prevent backflow. The capillaries, the smallest vessels, directly serve cellular needs and their fine walls allow the easy passage of substances between the tissues and the blood stream.

The walls of arteries and veins have three layers: the tunica interna, tunica media and tunica externa. Capillary walls consist only of endothelium and sparse basal lamina.[3]

ACTIVITY

- Using an anatomy and physiology textbook of your choice, revise the following:
  - anatomy and physiology of the heart
  - the coronary circulation
  - electrical conduction in the heart
  - the major veins and arteries of the systemic circulation.

- Draw a diagram of the heart and label the following structures:
  - left and right atria, left and right ventricles, inferior and superior vena cava, aorta, mitral valve, tricuspid valve, pulmonary valve, pulmonary arteries, pulmonary veins, endocardium, myocardium, pericardium.

- Check your diagram using an anatomy and physiology textbook (e.g. *Human Anatomy and Physiology*[3]).

- If you prefer, an online tutorial on the anatomy and physiology of the heart is available at: http://www.le.ac.uk/pathology/teach/va/anatomy/case1/frmst1.html

- An online exploration of the heart is available at: http://sln.fi.edu/biosci/biosci.html

- Cardiovascular anatomy quizzes are available at: http://www.gen.umn.edu/faculty_staff/jensen/1135/webanatomy/wa_cvs/default.htm

---

DRIVERS FOR CARE

The White Paper *Saving Lives: Our Healthier Nation* aimed to improve health and reduce inequalities in health.[5] Social disadvantage is inextricably linked to the risk of premature death, and the target for CHD was to 'reduce the death rate from CHD and stroke and related diseases in people under 75 years by at least two-fifths by 2010 – saving up to 200,000 lives in total'.[5]

The National Service Framework (NSF) for CHD issued in 2000 was one of the first NSFs.[2] CHD was an early target, not only because there is better evidence for the prevention, diagnosis and treatment of CHD than for many other major diseases, but also because evidence indicated that research findings were being incompletely and variably applied in practice. CHD exemplifies inequalities in health and a countrywide variation in services was evident.[2]

The NSF is a 10-year plan to reduce premature deaths from CHD and promote faster and fairer access to high-quality services. It aims to reduce inconsistency in access to services, improve the overall quality of care, improve outcomes and ultimately improve the health of the nation.

Twelve standards have been set, covering the prevention, diagnosis and treatment of CHD.

The National Institute for Health and Clinical Excellence (NICE) is an independent organisation responsible for providing national guidance on

---

ACTIVITY

A survey carried out in 2004 found that one person in three of those with heart disease also has undiagnosed diabetes.[17]

How do you approach screening for diabetes among patients with, or at high risk of, CHD?

In the course of your consultations with diabetic patients, consider how you increase patient awareness of the role of cardiovascular risk factor management in maintaining health.

treatments and care for people using the NHS in England and Wales. NICE has developed several guidelines and tools to support the care of patients with CHD.

The new GMS (nGMS) contract was implemented in April 2004.[6] The contract makes recommendations for service provision in ten disease areas, and sets out the points available to be earned by practices that implement them. Earning points translates into monetary achievement, with payments related to targets. The management of CHD attracts the highest number of points (121 of the 550 clinical points available), and so has the potential to bring GP practices the greatest cost benefits.[7] Adding the points available for diabetes and hypertension increases the total to 59% of the points available in relation to clinical indicators.[8]

Practice nurses are pivotal to successful delivery of the nGMS contract, and nurse-led CHD clinics leading to improved medical and lifestyle management are a successful strategy.[9]

THE CARDIAC COLLABORATIVE

The Cardiac Collaborative operates as part of the NHS Modernisation Agency. There are 30 local programmes operating across England, and project managers work with local clinical teams to redesign and improve cardiac services.[10] Each CHD Collaborative operates six projects focused around the NSF, namely:

- secondary prevention
- acute myocardial infarction
- angina
- heart failure
- cardiac surgery
- cardiac rehabilitation.

The White Paper, *Choosing Health: Making Healthy Choices Easier*[11] builds upon *Saving Lives: Our Healthier Nation*[5] and sets out key principles

---

EVALUATION ACTIVITY

Reflect critically on the provision of care for high-risk groups, taking into account the influence of the new GMS Contract and the NSF.

LEARNING POINTS

- CHD is the leading cause of death in the UK
- A raft of national drivers for care exists to support practice in CHD management
- Social disadvantage contributes to premature death
- Practice nurses are pivotal in providing preventive care to patients at risk of CHD
- Women are emerging as a group with serious CHD risks and can suffer from inequality of care
- People with diabetes are two to four times more likely to develop cardiovascular disease

---

to support healthier and informed choices. Health is inextricably linked to lifestyle, and the strategies aim to shape the commercial and cultural drivers of lifestyle.

REFERENCES

1. British Heart Foundation. Coronary Heart Disease Statistics. Factsheet. London: BHF, 2004. Available at: http://www.heartstats.org
2. Department of Health. National Service Framework for Coronary Heart Disease. London: HMSO, 2000.
3. Marieb EN. Human Anatomy and Physiology, 6th edn. Harlow: Pearson Education, 2004.
4. The Virtual Autopsy. Cardiovascular System Anatomy and Physiology. Available at: http://www.le.ac.uk/pathology/teach/va/anatomy/case1/frmst1.html
5. Department of Health. Saving Lives: Our Healthier Nation. London: HMSO, 1999.
6. NHS Executive. General Medical Services Contract. London: HMSO, 2004.
7. Pharmafocus 2004. OTC Statins: Lifesaver or Lifestyle? Available at: http://www.pharmafocus.com/cda/focusH/1,2109,22-0-0-SEP_2004-focus_feature_detail-0-244856,-00.html
8. NHS Modernisation Agency. Service Improvement. Coronary Heart Disease Secondary Prevention Workstream: Planning Workshops – September 2004 (Core Presentation – Afternoon). Available at: http://www.modern.nhs.uk/scripts/default.asp?site_id=23&id=26258
9. Murchie P, Campbell NC, Ritchie LD, Simpson JA, Thain J. Secondary prevention clinics for coronary heart disease: four year follow up of a randomised controlled trial in primary care. BMJ 2003; 326: 84.
10. NHS Modernisation Agency. Coronary Heart Disease Collaborative, 2003. Available at: http://www.modern.nhs.uk/scripts/default.asp?site_id=23&id=11236
11. Department of Health. Choosing Health: Making Healthier Choices Easier. London: HMSO, 2004.
12. Lindsay GM. risk factor assessment. In: Lindsay GM, Gaw A (eds), Coronary Heart Disease Prevention. A Handbook for the Health Care Team. London: Churchill Livingstone, 1997.
13. British Heart Foundation. Factfile: Coronary Heart Disease in Women. London: BHF, 2003.
14. British Heart Foundation. Factfile: Family History of Coronary Heart Disease in Primary Care. London: BHF, 2003.
15. British Heart Foundation. British Heart Foundation Launches New Health Services for Ethnic Minorities [press release]. London: BHF, 2002. Available at: http://www.bhf.org.uk
16. Johnston DW. The current status of the coronary-prone behaviour pattern. J Sociol Med 1993; 86: 406–409.
17. European Society of Cardiology. Diabetes and the Heart. Survey, 2004. Available at: http://www.diabetes.org.uk

Chapter 23

CARDIOVASCULAR DISEASE

Primary prevention of coronary heart disease

Sarah Kraszewski

LEARNING OBJECTIVES

After reading this chapter you will be able to:

- demonstrate an awareness of key effective interventions towards primary prevention of coronary heart disease (CHD)
- discuss strategies to offer primary prevention to the general population
- understand the benefits and limitations of risk calculation in CHD
- be aware of several available CHD risk calculators and be able to apply their use to practice
- be aware of the application in practice of the CHD National Service Framework

Standards One and Two (Box 23.1) and Chapter One of the National Service Framework for Coronary Heart Disease[1] (NSF for CHD) address the issues of primary prevention of CHD in the population. Key effective interventions include reducing smoking, promoting healthy eating, promoting physical activity and reducing overweight and obesity.

SMOKING

Smoking is the most common avoidable cause of ill health and premature death in the UK.

BOX 23.1   The NSF for CHD: recommendations on primary prevention
Standard one The NHS and partner agencies should develop, implement and monitor policies that reduce the prevalence of coronary risk factors in the population, and reduce inequalities in risks of developing heart disease
Standard two The NHS and partner agencies should contribute to a reduction in the prevalence of smoking in the local population

platelet production increase the risk of clotting. As a result of these effects, smokers are at higher risk of developing atherosclerotic disease.[2]

One of the most effective interventions a health professional can make is to support a patient in quitting smoking. Smoking-cessation services that provide behavioural support and advice are effective in helping smokers to quit. A structured programme, run by specialists, that entails regular contact over a period of at least 4 weeks can double the success rates even in those not using NRT or buproprion (Zyban). These medications can quadruple the success rate compared with that achieved in would-be quitters not using them.[3]

Individuals in all sections of society are affected, by smoking themselves or by the effects of passive smoking.

Inhaling tobacco smoke affects the heart and blood vessels. The smoker's heart rate rises, nicotine causes blood pressure to rise, constriction of blood vessels increases the work of the heart and carbon monoxide reduces the ability of the blood to carry oxygen. Additionally, smoking tends to raise blood lipids and alter the HDL/LDL ratio. Raised levels of fibrinogen and increased

OBESITY

Obesity and overweight increase the risk of CHD in addition to that of other major diseases. Almost 24 million adults in the UK are overweight or obese, and rising obesity levels in children are likely to shorten life expectancy. The increasing levels of overweight and obesity have prompted national initiatives to tackle the problem.[4]

For those who are overweight (body mass index (BMI) > 25) or obese (BMI > 30), a weight loss of 10% will offer significant health benefits.[1] Individuals with a central pattern of obesity ('apple-shaped' rather than 'pear-shaped') are at higher risk of cardiovascular mortality and of developing hypertension and type 2 diabetes.[5] Losing weight can reduce blood pressure and levels of circulating LDL cholesterol and triglycerides, while increasing HDL cholesterol and reducing insulin resistance.

Ideally, individuals should maintain their weight within the normal range for their age, height and sex. The National Institute for Health and Clinical Excellence (NICE) plans to publish guidance on the prevention, identification, management and treatment of obesity in 2007. Some patients will require drug therapy to supplement dietary action for weight loss.

ACTIVITY
Carry out an audit of smoking-cessation interventions (based on the next 20 patients you see or observe).
Has a smoking status been recorded in the past year or at all?
If the patient is a smoker or ex-smoker, what evidence is in the notes of intervention on the part of the health professional?
What opportunities are you finding to talk about smoking cessation with patients?
Do you always ask a patient their smoking status?
If not, why might this be? Explore your own attitudes to asking people about smoking.

Two prescription drugs, which work in different ways, are licensed in the UK for the treatment of obesity: sibutramine (Reductil) and orlistat (Xenical).[6]

ACTIVITY

Reflect upon how you discuss the issue of weight with patients.

How do you support patients wanting to lose weight?

What resources are available at your surgery?

What means of assessing body fat, other than BMI calculation, are available?

Review the clinical indications and contraindications for the two drugs that can be prescribed for the management of obesity.

Can you identify patients for whom these might be suitable therapies?

What monitoring is required?

PHYSICAL ACTIVITY

Sedentary modern lifestyles increase cardio-vascular risks, and few adults and children are sufficiently active to benefit their health.[4] The benefits of regular physical activity include lowering the risk of CHD and stroke, hypertension, overweight and obesity, type 2 diabetes, osteoporosis, some cancers, dyslipidaemia and depressed mood.

Adults should build up to 30 minutes of moderate activity (activity that makes an individual feel warm and breathe faster, but does not prevent them from holding a conversation) 5 days of the week. The exercise does not have to be taken all in one go – 10 minutes of activity three times a day is just as effective.[7] Successful interventions include home-based programmes, unsupervised informal exercise and frequent professional contact, with walking as the promoted mode of exercise.

ACTIVITY

There are many local initiatives to support people in becoming more active, such as exercise referral programmes and guided walks. Contact your local PCT to find out what initiatives are available for your patients.

How might pedometers assist your patients in increasing their activity levels?

HEALTHY EATING

The aim of promoting healthy eating is to encourage consumption of a balanced diet by everyone in the community. The current emphasis is on eating more fruit and vegetables and starchy foods such as bread, rice, pasta, potatoes and unrefined grains and more fish (especially oily fish), a smaller proportion of foods containing fat and saturated fat, and less salt.[8] Eating healthily can both reduce the risk of developing CHD and increase the chances of survival after diagnosis of CHD.

The Mediterranean diet is thought to contain cardioprotective elements.[9] Individuals should aim to eat at least five portions of fruit and vegetables a day, increase antioxidant consumption, reduce the total amount of dietary fat and replace saturated and trans fats with mono-unsaturated and polyunsaturated fats to improve the HDL/LDL ratio.

ACTIVITY

How do patients access dietetic advice in your practice?

What training does the practice nurse need to fulfil this function?

Useful patient information leaflets in a variety of languages are available from the British Heart Foundation. Ensure you have available for all patients a supply of appropriate leaflets.

The consumption of omega-3 fatty acids (available in fish and plant sources) is beneficial.[9] Salt consumption should be reduced. Moderate alcohol consumption (1–2 units a day) may have a protective function, but excessive consumption may lead to hypertension and weight gain.

Other general advice includes increasing fibre intake; soluble fibre may help reduce cholesterol. Particular attention needs to be paid to the diet of school children and those in low-income and ethnic groups.

LIPID MANAGEMENT

People whose circulating total cholesterol level is above 5 mmol/l and who are at high risk of CHD should be offered lipid-lowering therapy. Dietary modification should be discussed with the patient, and if necessary treatment with a statin started.

The consumption of 2–3 g/day of plant sterols/stanols has been shown to reduce LDL cholesterol levels by 9–20%.[10] Treatment aims to lower total cholesterol by 20–25% or to below 5 mmol/l, whichever is lower, and LDL cholesterol by 30% or to below 3 mmol/l.[1] The Heart Protection Study found that lowering cholesterol from 4 mmol/l to 3 mmol/l reduced CHD risks by 25%.[11] These findings are not reflected in the NSF or current NICE guidelines. NICE plans to publish guidelines on lipid lowering in 2007.

RISK CALCULATION

Effective interventions can decrease CHD risk. To target people appropriately, you must consider the nature and level of risk. CHD risk cannot be calculated on the basis of single risk factors. The Framingham study showed how CHD risk increases in the presence of multiple risk factors.[12] A variety of risk calculators, mostly based on the Framingham study, has been developed to assess CHD risk, and practice computer systems often incorporate these.

The British Hypertension Society (BHS) and others have produced updated recommendations and replaced assessment of CHD risk with that of cardiovascular disease (CVD) risk, so as to include patients at risk from stroke. A CVD threshold of less than 20% approximately equates with a CHD risk of more than 15% over 10 years.[13] Simplified risk assessment charts (Figure 23.1) now have three age bands and none for people with type 2 diabetes, who should be assessed as if they have established CHD.[14]

It is important to note the limitations of the charts; they address only six variables and are intended as a guide, not a directive.[14] The assessment may underestimate risk in some groups, such as in those with family history, and overestimate risk in others, such as in young people with diabetes.[14]

Those with diagnosed heart or vascular disease do not require a risk calculation, as they are known to be at high risk for further events (30% over 10 years is considered high risk). Those with a risk of between 15% and 30% over 10 years will also require intensive management.

The following section should be read bearing in mind the latest recommendations from the BHS on CVD risk, and the results from the Heart Protection Study on lipid lowering, neither of which are incorporated into the CHD NSF. NICE guidance scheduled for publication in 2007 will provide further clarification on the issues of lipid management.

For individuals whose 10-year CHD risk is calculated to be more than 30% but who have not been diagnosed with CHD or other occlusive vascular disease, the NSF recommends offering personalised advice and information on reducing modifiable risk factors. Action to modify risk factors includes smoking cessation (including the use of NRT or buproprion), improved diet, increased physical activity, weight reduction, reduced alcohol consumption and control of diabetes mellitus.

In addition, advice and treatment should be given to maintain blood pressure below 140/85 noting that the presence of diabetes mellitus or

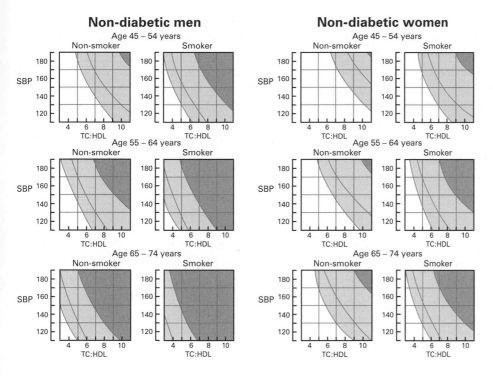

Figure 23.1 Risk assessment charts: examples.

proteinurea or microalbuminurea will necessitate tighter control. Low-dose aspirin is recommended for the over-50s, and those with risks > 15% or with diabetes or target-organ damage.[15] An alternative antiplatelet agent will be necessary for anyone hypersensitive to aspirin.

With regard to blood lipids, the aim should be to reduce serum total cholesterol by 20–25% or to below 5 mmol/l, whichever is lower, by means of appropriate dietetic advice and statin therapy. Serum LDL cholesterol should be lowered by 30% or to below 3 mmol/l, whichever is lower. People with diabetes should be supported to maintain meticulous control of blood pressure and glucose.[1]

For those with a 10-year CHD risk of 15–30%, the above advice applies, but with modified advice regarding lipids. The NSF recommends offering statins and dietary advice to lower serum total cholesterol below 5 mmol/l to people with diabetes, and those with a familial dyslipidaemia. Otherwise, offer diet and lifestyle advice, and follow up every 3–5 years. Total cholesterol greater than 7.8 mmol/l must raise the issue of possible familial dyslipidaemia.[9]

ACTIVITY

Select 10 adult patients from the age–sex register (take a mixture of ages and sexes). Review their notes and consider their risk factors. Note any factors excluding use of the charts. Calculate their risk for CVD using risk calculators. Risk assessment charts are printed at the back of the BNF. Alternatively, several are available to view or download from the Internet:

- Framingham function for risk estimation: http://www.cvhealth.ed.ac.uk/index.html
- Joint British Societies Cardiovascular Disease Risk Prediction Chart: http://www.bhsoc.org/ Cardiovascular_Risk_Charts_and_Calculators. htm
- A suite of algorithms and risk prediction tools: http://www.medal.org
- UK Prospective Diabetes Study Risk Engine, risk in people with type 2 diabetes: http://www.dtu.ox.ac.uk

How did your intuitive estimation of their risks compare with the calculated figure?

For individuals with a CHD risk calculated to be more than 15% over 10 years, most will not need treatment but should be offered information and advice on modifiable risk factors and lifestyle. Their 10-year risk of CHD should be reassessed in 3–5 years.[1]

The latest BHS guidelines recommend statin therapy for primary prevention in all people with a 10-year CVD risk more than 20%, and targets of reducing total cholesterol by 25% or to more than 4 mmol/l, and LDL by 30% or to less than 2 mmol/l.

The financial impact of prescribing for every individual who falls into this category would be immense. Simvastatin 10 mg is available for purchase over-the-counter to people with a 10–15% CHD risk over 10 years. This includes all men over 55 years, plus men aged 45–55 and women over 55 who have a family history of CHD, are smokers, obese, centrally obese or of south Asian descent.[16]

The variation in the published guidelines represents the evolving evidence base; each patient should be individually assessed, and treatment targeted appropriately.

HRT in menopausal women has not been shown to be of benefit in primary prevention of CHD, and some studies have shown it to be associated with slight increases in CHD rates.[9]

HRT should not be used for prevention of CHD and stopping it should be considered after a cardiovascular event.[17]

CONCLUSION

Primary prevention of CHD entails assessment of risk and health education to support patients in deciding how to modify risky behaviours. The practice nurse is ideally placed to undertake this role.

EVALUATION ACTIVITY

Evaluate how successfully the practice strategies are in promoting primary preventtion of CHD.

What services are being offered to patients in accordance with national policy?

LEARNING POINTS

- Risk calculators have replaced intuition in calculating risk, but have limitations
- CHD risk calculation has been replaced with CVD risk
- Key effective interventions include smoking cessation, weight management, increasing physical activity and healthy eating
- NICE is scheduled to publish guidance on the use of statins in primary and secondary CHD prevention in 2007
- The practice nurse can support patients in modifying risky behaviours

---

ACTIVITY

Using your CHD disease register, select 20 patients assessed as having a CHD risk of 15–30%.

Review the interventions to see whether all modifiable risk factors are being adequately addressed.

REFERENCES

1. Department of Health. National Service Framework for Coronary Heart Disease. London: The Stationery Office, 2000.
2. ASH. Smoking, the Heart and Circulation. Fact Sheet No. 6, 2004. Available at: http://www.ash.org.uk
3. West R, McNeill A, Raw M. Smoking cessation guidelines for health professionals: an update. Thorax 2000; 55: 987–999.
4. Department of Health. Choosing Health: Making Healthier Choices Easier. London: The Stationery Office, 2004.

5. Glenny A, O'Meara S (eds). The Prevention and Treatment of Obesity. Effective Health Care 1997; 3(2). York: NHS Centre for Reviews and Dissemination.

6. Mead M. Drugs for obesity. Practice Nurse 2004; 28(10 September): 64–67.

7. British Heart Foundation. Get Active booklet, 2004. Available at: http://www.bhf.org.uk

8. Committee on Medical Aspects of Food Policy (COMA). Nutritional Aspects of Cardiovascular Disease. London: HMSO, 1994.

9. Prodigy Guidance, 2003. Coronary Heart Disease: Risk Identification and Management. http://www.prodigy. nhs.uk/guidance.asp?gt=CHD%20risk%20%20identify %20and%20manage

10. British Heart Foundation. Cholesterol Lowering: Stanols and Sterols. Factfile, 2002. Available at: http://www.bhf.org.uk

11. Heart Protection Study Collaborative Group. MRC/BHF heart protection study of cholesterol lowering with simvastatin in 20,536 high-risk individuals: a randomised placebo-controlled trial. Lancet 2002; 360: 7–22.

12. Lindsay GM. risk factor assessment. In: Lindsay GM, Gaw A (eds), Coronary Heart Disease Prevention. A Handbook for the Health Care Team. London: Churchill Livingstone, 1997.

13. British Hypertension Society Guidelines Working Party. Guidelines for the management of hypertension: report of the Fourth Working Party of the British Hypertension Society 2004. J Hum Hypertens 2004; 18: 139–185.

14. British Heart Foundation. Updated Guidelines on Cardiovascular Disease Risk Assessment. Factfile, 2004. Available at: http://www.bhf.org.uk

15. Guidelines for Management of Hypertension: Report of the Fourth Working Party of the British Hypertension Society (BHS IV), 2004. J Hum Hypertens 2004; 18: 139–185.

16. Blenkinsop J, Gathoga L, O'Connel K, et al. OTC simvastatin supply – what education do pharmacists want? Pharm J 2004; 273(7 August): 191–193.

17. Committee on the Safety of Medicines. New product information for hormone replacement therapy. Curr Problems Pharmacovigilance 2002; 28(April): 1–2.

Chapter 24

CARDIOVASCULAR DISEASE

Secondary prevention of coronary heart disease

Sarah Kraszewski

LEARNING OBJECTIVES

After reading this chapter you will be able to:

- describe the common presentations of coronary heart disease (CHD)
- discuss strategies for offering secondary prevention to those diagnosed with CHD
- discuss the organisation of CHD management within primary care
- reflect on the relationship between primary care and acute services
- outline the content of a chronic disease management appointment for a patient with CHD

This chapter deals with secondary prevention of coronary heart disease (CHD) and the organisation and delivery of treatment in primary care.

Coronary heart disease may manifest itself as angina pectoris, myocardial infarction, congestive heart failure or sudden death.[1]

ANGINA PECTORIS

Angina pectoris is caused by reversible myocardial ischaemia, which is usually the result of atherosclerotic disease in the coronary arteries. Chest pain and tightness may radiate to one or both arms, to the throat and to the back. Symptoms may be brought on by activity or emotion, or may occur at rest. Stable angina is characterised by chest pain following exertion and relieved by rest. Unstable angina describes prolonged episodes of severe angina, increasingly frequent angina, or angina at rest.[2]

The symptoms of angina may be confused with those of other conditions, such as musculoskeletal pain, gastro-oesophageal reflux, pericarditis and pulmonary embolism.[1] Rapid-access, chest pain clinics are available at many hospitals to provide prompt assessment of patients with suspected angina.

ACTIVITY

Locate your local rapid-access chest pain clinic and find out how patients are referred to the service.

Arrange a visit, so that you understand the patient journey.

ACUTE MYOCARDIAL INFARCTION

Acute myocardial infarction (AMI) results when prolonged myocardial ischaemia leads to development of a localised area of necrosis in the myocardium.[1] AMI symptoms are listed in Box 24.1. If the heart is not tipped into fibrillation, and damage to the heart muscle is not too massive, the patient may survive AMI.[3]

The initial cause of reduced blood flow to the myocardium may be an intracoronary thrombus associated with plaque fissure, haemorrhage into an atheromatous plaque, or platelet aggregation in the presence of atheroma and possible thrombus.[1] Severe hypotension may reduce coronary artery flow and cause infarction. Pain from an AMI is not relieved by nitrates or rest, and can be prolonged. Some elderly patients may experience a 'silent' infarction and present with heart failure.

BOX 24.1 Symptoms associated with acute myocardial infarction[1]

- Severe crushing central chest pain
- Dyspnoea
- Syncope
- Cold sweat
- Pallor
- Nausea
- Sudden death

THROMBOLYSIS

The term 'thrombolysis' refers to the use of clot-dissolving drugs that, if administered soon after AMI, can reduce the risk of death and disability. The sooner they are administered, the better the outcome (Box 24.2), and in some parts of the UK paramedics are trained to administer them. Aspirin reduces clot formation and cuts the risk of death by about one-quarter.[4]

The number of patients receiving life-saving thrombolysis within 30 minutes of hospital arrival rose from 59% in April 2002 to 81% in December 2003.[5] Patients often delay calling for help for up to an hour,[6] and call-to-needle times are improved by having patients with chest pain dial 999. A raft of service improvements has evolved through the Cardiac Collaborative work to simplify the patient journey and reduce delays.[7] Guidance on thrombolysis can be found at http://www.nice.org.uk.

BOX 24.2 The NSF for coronary heart disease: thrombolysis[4]

Standard 6
People thought to be suffering from a heart attack should be assessed professionally and, if indicated, receive aspirin. Thrombolysis should be given within 60 minutes of calling for professional help

Seven hundred automated external defibrillators have been installed in 110 public places around the UK, to help increase the chance of survival for the 12,000 people who suffer cardiac arrest in a public place each year.[8]

ACTIVITY

As many as 50% of all deaths from acute myocardial infarction (AMI) occur within 2 hours of onset, and most of these deaths occur outside of hospital.[1] Many patients are worried about dialling 999 and 'wasting people's time'.

Reflect on how you discuss with patients the issues of signs and symptoms of AMI and how to summon help, and how to transfer the important message about prompt treatment.

HEART FAILURE

Heart failure (Boxes 24.3 and 24.4) is a clinical condition where the heart fails to pump into the circulation sufficient blood for tissue metabolic needs. Dyspnoea is a predominant feature of heart failure, because of engorgement of the pulmonary vessels and failure of the left ventricle.[1]

An average GP (list size 2,000) will see about 20 people with heart failure each year.[9] The increased

---

BOX 24.3   The NSF for coronary heart disease: heart failure[4]

Standard 11
Doctors should arrange for people with suspected heart failure to be offered appropriate investigations (e.g. electrocardiography, echocardiography) that will confirm or refute the diagnosis. For those in whom heart failure is confirmed, its cause should be identified –the treatments most likely both to relieve symptoms and to reduce the risk of death should be offered

---

ACTIVITY

Primary care teams are required to offer regular review to people with established heart failure.[4]

How does your practice structure the care of patients diagnosed with heart failure?

Contact your local heart failure specialist nurse to establish how you can work collaboratively to improve patient care.

What further training might the practice nurse require to work with this group of patients?

---

prevalence of heart failure is a result both of the increased number of people surviving AMI with residual cardiac damage and of an ageing population.[4] Other causes of heart failure include hypertension, cardiomyopathy, diseases of the heart valves, congenital heart disease, some endocrine disorders and, rarely, anaemia.[10]

Prognosis with heart failure is poor, with a high risk of sudden death,[4] and heart failure is a debilitating disease. Patients cared for by specialist nurses may have an improved quality of life and survival rates.[11] Cardiac rehabilitation, palliative care and long-term social support may be necessary.

Early diagnosis enables the condition to be controlled with the right combination of drugs and lifestyle changes. An echocardiogram is recommended to confirm diagnosis. Treatment with ACE inhibitors improves prognosis and relieves symptoms;[4] loop and thiazide diuretics

---

BOX 24.4   Symptoms of chronic heart failure[12]

- Shortness of breath on exertion
- Decreased exercise tolerance (often simply 'fatigue')
- Paroxysmal nocturnal dyspnoea
- Orthopnoea
- Ankle swelling

may be considered for those with signs of fluid overload, and beta-blockers are indicated for those with stable heart failure (unless the individual has contraindications). Spironolactone, digoxin, and angiotensin-II receptor antagonists may be indicated for particular patients. Treatment should be started under specialist supervision unless the GP has particular expertise in this area.[12]

ATRIAL FIBRILLATION

Atrial fibrillation (AF) is a common arrhythmia associated with CHD, heart failure, valvular disease or hypertension, but may also exist in patients with normal hearts.[13] AF may reduce cardiac output and symptoms may include palpitations, tiredness, fatigue or dizziness. Not all patients report symptoms. The pulse should be checked during the consultation and any irregularity followed up with a 12-lead electrocardiogram (ECG). AF is a significant risk factor for stroke. Treatment may involve anticoagulant therapy, anti-arrhythmic drugs and electrical cardioversion for suitable patients. The National Institute for Health and Clinical Excellence is developing a guideline (due in 2006).

personalised advice and information on reducing modifiable risk factors (Box 24.5). Measures might include smoking cessation (including the use of NRT or bupropion), attention to diet, increased physical activity, weight control, moderation of alcohol consumption, and control of diabetes mellitus.

In addition, advice and treatment should be given to maintain blood pressure below 140/85,[14] noting that the presence of diabetes mellitus or proteinurea or microalbuminurea will necessitate tighter control (130/80).[14] Low-dose aspirin, 75 mg/day, is recommended, with an alternative antiplatelet agent for those hypersensitive to aspirin.

Statins and dietary advice will aim to lower serum total cholesterol by 20–25% or to reduce it to below 5.0 mmol/l, whichever would result in the lower level. (Serum low-density lipoprotein cholesterol should be lowered by 30% or reduced to below 3.0 mmol/l, whichever would result in the lower level.) The latest BHS recommendations for people with hypertension complicated by diagnosed cardiovascular disease recommend statin therapy irrespective of baseline levels.[14]

Patients with left ventricular dysfunction should be treated with ACE inhibitors. Beta-

---

ACTIVITY

How is warfarin monitoring organised in your practice?

Where do the patients attend for their blood tests, and how do they receive their results?

What potential can you see for the improvement of services in your practice?

SECONDARY PREVENTION

Individuals who have been diagnosed with CHD, or other occlusive vascular disease, should receive

---

BOX 24.5   The NSF for coronary heart disease: secondary prevention

Standard 3
General practitioners and primary care teams should identify all people with established cardiovascular disease, and offer them comprehensive advice and appropriate treatment to reduce their risks

Standard 4
General practitioners and primary health care teams should identify all people at significant risk of cardiovascular disease but who have not yet developed symptoms, and offer them appropriate advice and treatment to reduce their risks

---

ACTIVITY

Patients with established coronary heart disease are likely to be on multiple medications.

For the following medications, how would you explain to the patient the mode of action, benefits and potential side-effects?

What monitoring might be required for individual medications?

– Aspirin
– Beta-blockers
– ACE inhibitors
– Nitrates
– Glyceryl trinitrate (GTN)
– Calcium-channel blockers
– Statins
– Diuretics
– Warfarin

BOX 24.6   The NSF for coronary heart disease: cardiac rehabilitation

Standard 12

NHS trusts should put in place agreed protocols/systems of care so that, before leaving hospital, people admitted to hospital because of coronary heart disease are invited to participate in a multidisciplinary programme of secondary prevention and cardiac rehabilitation. The aim of the programme will be to reduce their risk of subsequent cardiac problems and to promote their return to a full and normal life

---

ACTIVITY

Review the care of 20 patients who have received revascularisation surgery or suffered AMI. How many have received cardiac rehabilitation?

How does the practice follow up patients discharged from hospital to ensure an opportunity for rehabilitation is available?

Contact your local cardiac rehabilitation nurses and, if possible, arrange to visit the programme.

Contact staff at a local coronary care unit (CCU) and, if possible, arrange a visit to the ward.

---

blockers and spironolactone may also be added. Angiotensin-II receptor antagonists may benefit those intolerant of ACE inhibitors. Following a myocardial infarction, beta-blockers and ACE inhibitors are indicated.

People over 60 years of age with atrial fibrillation require warfarin or aspirin, depending on individual risks of stroke. Those with diabetes mellitus require meticulous control of blood glucose and blood pressure.[4, 15]

CARDIAC REHABILITATION

A more intensive approach to understanding the nature of CHD and its treatment helps individuals to achieve lifestyle changes, regain confidence and return to as normal a life as possible. Only one-third of patients discharged after AMI or coronary surgery currently receive rehabilitation,[14] and the NSF sets a target of 85% (Box 24.6). To improve this, the BHF is setting up 40 community-based rehabilitation programmes to support the recovery of this group of patients.

PSYCHOLOGICAL IMPACT OF CHD

Patients with CHD may manifest signs of depression and anxiety. They may worry about heart attacks or the success of surgery, or fear dying. The implications of their illness for work and relationships may cause additional worry.

Long-term anxiety and depression will affect the quality and duration of life. It is important to make time for people to talk to you about their feelings and emotions. Men may be embarrassed to talk about their worries concerning the effect on their sexual relationships. The nurse should offer time and empathy, and understand the

---

ACTIVITY

How can the practice nurse offer psychological support to patients and their families?

You might like to consider:
- information giving
- listening skills
- support agencies
- the patient journey: coordination of services
- screening and referral
- concordance.

---

psychological impact of being diagnosed with cardiovascular disease.

EXPERT PATIENTS PROGRAMME

The Expert Patients Programme (EPP) offers people with long-term conditions opportunities to build on their own knowledge by learning new skills to support living with their condition.

ACTIVITY

Setting up a CHD clinic
- You are asked to set up a regular clinic to review patients with, or at high risk of, CHD:
  - What factors might you need to consider when planning your sessions?
- A disease register is a means to organise disease management more effectively and efficiently so that clinical outcomes and performance can be measured:
  - How might a practice identify patients with CHD to enable their details to be added to the register?
  - How are new patients identified and added?
- How might you facilitate a call-and-recall system? Why do you need one?
- How might you systematically identify your at-risk patients?
- How will you invite patients to attend?
- How might you approach non-responders?

The NSF for CHD contains, in Chapter 2, an example of a protocol for the prevention of CHD in practice.
- What training might the practice nurse require so as to be able to offer this service?
- What topics might you expect to discuss with your patients during a consultation?
- What blood tests/investigations might you require? How can you organise these in advance of the consultation to make best use of your and the patient's time?

The care of the patient with CHD will require a multidisciplinary teamwork approach, and shared care between primary and acute care.
- Which health professionals are likely to be involved in the delivery of care?
- How can administrative staff support the service?
- How can communication between team members be facilitated?

Many general practices rely on computer systems.
- Reflect on your own skills in information technology.
- What further training might you require to use the systems to their best advantage?
- How can the computer system support your clinic organisation and audit processes?

A multidisciplinary team approach is necessary for effective care of this patient group. The practice nurse is a key member of the team and can provide regular review and coordinate the patient's care.

ACTIVITY

Contact your local PCT to find out how they are supporting the Expert Patients Programme (EPP).

Ensure you have a supply of EPP leaflets in the surgery for patients to take away with them.

LEARNING POINTS

- Patient information on CHD should include when to call 999
- Patients with CHD may be on multiple medications
- Advice on modifiable risky behaviours is a key intervention
- Systematic organisation in practice is key to the successful delivery of services
- Currently, many patients do not receive cardiac rehabilitation because of a shortage of services
- Patients with heart failure can achieve a better quality of life through referral to specialist nurses and services

---

Further information is available at http://www.expertpatients.nhs.uk.

ORGANISATION OF CHD MANAGEMENT

Systematic care is key in strategies for the management of primary and secondary prevention. According to the NSF, this should be through:

- routine consultation structured by a specific protocol
- nurse-led specialist CHD clinics
- nurse-led services at PCT level.

It is necessary to identify all patients at risk and those with established disease, and establish a validated practice register. The register will enable the practice to plan and prioritise care through the use of a call-and-recall system and protocols. The register, and a team approach to use of correct Read codes and computerised management plans,

---

EVALUATION ACTIVITY

Reflect critically on the current care of people with heart disease in your practice.

Identify strengths and weaknesses in the organisational system and in clinical care.

---

will facilitate audit and help the practice earn CHD quality points under the new GMS contract. Patient-held record cards can help coordinate team care and give patients ownership of their disease.

REFERENCES

1. Lorimar AR. Coronary heart disease. In: Lindsay GM, Gaw A (eds), Coronary Heart Disease Prevention: A Handbook for the Health Care Team. Edinburgh: Churchill Livingstone, 1997.
2. Scottish Intercollegiate Guidelines Network. Management of Stable Angina. Clinical Guideline 51. Edinburgh: SIGN, 2001. Available at: http://www.sign.ac.uk
3. Marieb EN. Human Anatomy and Physiology, 6th edn. Harlow: Pearson Education, 2004.
4. Department of Health. National Service Framework for Coronary Heart Disease. London: HMSO, 2000.
5. Petersen S, Peto V, Rayner M. 2004 Coronary Heart Disease Statistics. London: British Heart Foundation, 2004. Available at: http://www.heartstats.org
6. Leslie WS, Urie A, Hooper J, Morrison CE. Delay in calling for help during myocardial infarction: reasons for the delay and subsequent pattern of accessing care. Heart 2000; 84: 137–141.
7. Department of Health. Review of Early Thrombolysis – Faster and Better Treatment for Heart Attack Patients. London: DoH, 2003. Available at: http://www.dh.gov.uk/PublicationsAndStatistics/ Publications/PublicationsPolicyAndGuidance/ PublicationsPolicyAndGuidanceArticle/fs/ en?CONTENT_ID=4008531&chk=Qq9TkY
8. Department of Health. Winning the War on Heart Disease – Progress Report. London: HMSO, 2004.
9. Eccles M, Freemantle N, Mason J. North of England evidence-based development project: guideline for

angiotensin converting enzyme inhibitors in primary care management of adults with symptomatic heart failure. BMJ 1998; 316: 1369–1375.

10. Netdoctor.co.uk. Encyclopedia of Diseases. Heart Failure. Available at: http://www.netdoctor.co.uk

11. British Heart Foundation. 'Hidden Killer' Places Huge Burden on UK [press release], 7 June 2002. Available at: http://www.bhf.org.uk

12. Prodigy Guidance 2004. Heart Failure. Available at: http://www.prodigy.nhs.uk

13. Simpson SH. Heart disease in primary care. In: Martin J, Lucas J (eds), Handbook of Practice Nursing, 3rd edn. Edinburgh: Churchill Livingstone, 2004.

14. Guidelines for Management of Hypertension: Report of the Fourth Working Party of the British Hypertension Society (BHS IV), 2004. J Hum Hypertens 2004; 18: 139–185.

15. National Institute for Health and Clinical Excellence. Prophylaxis for Patients who have Experienced a Myocardial Infarction. Inherited Clinical Guideline A. London: NICE, 2001. Available at: http://www.nice.org.uk

FURTHER INFORMATION

Action on Smoking and Health (ASH): http://www.ash.org.uk

British Heart Foundation: http://www.bhf.org.uk

Cardiac Collaboratives: http://www.modern.nhs.uk/scripts/default.asp?site_id=23

Department of Health: http://www.dh.gov.uk

Health Development Agency. Coronary Heart Disease: Guidance for Implementing the Preventive Aspects of the National Service Framework: http://www.publichealth.nice.org.uk/page.aspx?o=501951

National Electronic Library for Health Directory of Resources for CHD: http://www.nelh.nhs.uk

National Institute for Health and Clinical Excellence: http://www.nice.org.uk

Prodigy Guidance: http://www.prodigy.nhs.uk

Chapter 25

CARDIOVASCULAR DISEASE
Hypertension

Sarah Kraszewski

LEARNING OBJECTIVES

After reading this chapter you will be able to:

- discuss the incidence of hypertension in the UK
- define hypertension
- identify the causes of hypertension
- describe and undertake the correct technique for measurement of blood pressure
- be conversant with the limitations of the devices used for measurement
- describe the two sets of current guidelines on the management of hypertension
- describe health promotion and preventive care for people with hypertension
- describe the effects of hypertension on long-term health
- describe some of the common drug therapies

Hypertension is a major health issue affecting about a billion people worldwide, and has been identified by the World Health Organization as one of the most important preventable causes of premature morbidity and mortality.[1] It is often managed in primary care by GPs and practice nurses.

About 20% of middle-aged adults have a raised diastolic pressure of 90–109 mmHg. It is particularly common in the Afro-Caribbean population, where about 50% of people aged over 40 years have hypertension. People of south

Asian origin also have a high prevalence of both hypertension and type 2 diabetes.[2, 3]

There is a clear relationship between blood pressure and cardiovascular disease risk.[4] As a result, several important documents – *Saving Lives, Our Healthier Nation*, the National Service Framework for coronary heart disease, and the 2004 White Paper *Choosing Health: Making Healthier Choices Easier* – focus on strategies to support a reduction in blood pressure.[5-7]

Hypertensive patients with diagnosed coronary heart disease (CHD) or diabetes require management according to the relevant guidelines.

Raised blood pressure may be asymptomatic, and if left untreated the complications can be devastating.[8] Undertreatment is common. Up to half of diagnosed patients may not reach the recommended blood pressure targets.[8]

DEFINITION AND CLASSIFICATION

Hypertension can be described as a sustained high systemic arterial blood pressure, and is associated with a significant increase in the incidence of complications such as myocardial infarction or stroke.[9, 10] It is generally classified as either essential or secondary.

Essential hypertension, the most common form, is of unknown cause. Secondary hypertension, where a clear cause can be determined, affects fewer than 5% of cases.[9] It can be drug-induced or linked to other factors such as renal, endocrine and vascular disorders.

The classification system set out in Table 25.1 equates with those used by the European Society of Hypertension, the World Health Organization

TABLE 25.1   Classification of blood pressure levels[4]

Category	Systolic blood pressure (mmHg)	Diastolic blood pressure (mmHg)
Optimal blood pressure	< 120	80
Normal blood pressure	< 130	< 85
High–normal blood pressure	130–139	85–89
Grade 1 hypertension (mild)	140–159	90–99
Grade 2 hypertension (moderate)	160–179	100–109
Grade 3 hypertension (severe)	> 180	> 110
Isolated systolic hypertension (Grade 1)	140–159	< 90
Isolated systolic hypertension (Grade 2)	> 160	< 90

and the International Society of Hypertension, and is based on clinic blood pressure values. If a patient's systolic and diastolic readings fall into different categories, the higher value should be taken for classification.

PHYSIOLOGY

Blood pressure is a continuous variable that fluctuates widely throughout the day in response to physical and mental stress. It is determined by cardiac output and peripheral (systemic) vascular resistance (PVR):

Blood pressure = cardiac output × PVR

Thus blood pressure can be raised by increased cardiac output or peripheral resistance, or reduced by a fall in either.

Normal blood pressure is maintained by a combination of physiological mechanisms. The autonomic nervous system receives continual information from baroreceptors (pressure sensors) in the carotid sinus and aortic arch. The information is relayed to the vasomotor centre in the brainstem.

The parasympathetic nervous system responds to a drop in blood pressure by increasing the heart rate and causing venous and arterial vasoconstriction, mediated by beta receptors and alpha receptors, respectively.[15] Low blood pressure (hypotension) pulls fluid from the interstitial space into the circulation to restore the circulating volume. The fluid exchange that occurs across the capillary membrane and interstitial space is referred to as the capillary fluid shift mechanism.

Hormonal mechanisms also play a part in controlling the rise and fall of blood pressure, causing vasodilation, vasoconstriction and changes in blood volume.

Stimulation of the sympathetic nervous system causes release of adrenalin and noradrenaline from the adrenal medulla, increasing cardiac output and activating vasoconstriction.

Hypotension increases renin and angiotensin production in the kidney. Angiotensin is converted in the lung to angiotensin II, a potent vasoconstrictor. The presence of these hormones stimulates production of aldosterone from the adrenal cortex, decreasing urinary fluid and electrolyte loss from the body.

The kidneys' role in regulating blood pressure is to raise or lower blood volume through fluid output and secretion of hormones. The kidneys are particularly important for long-term control of blood pressure.

MEASURING BLOOD PRESSURE

Conventional sphygmomanometry was introduced by Riva-Rocci in 1896 and modified by Korotkoff in 1905. Directives on the disposal of mercury have prompted replacement of the traditional sphygmomanometer with semi-automated devices.

Diagnosis, monitoring and treatment depend on reliable measurement of blood pressure, so it is important to maintain skills and understand the influence of a variety of factors on the readings obtained. Doctors and nurses can show a surprising degree of inaccuracy in blood pressure measurement.[11] Poor technique can produce false readings, leading to unnecessary or inappropriate treatment and follow-up.

ACTIVITY

Factors that control blood pressure can be manipulated by drugs.

Choose an anatomy and physiology reference book and revise in greater detail the action of the sympathetic nervous system, the renin–angiotensin–aldosterone system, and the mechanisms of capillary fluid exchange and the kidney.

Consider how the drugs commonly used in hypertension may manipulate these mechanisms.

ACTIVITY

When did you last undertake training in blood pressure measurement? Revise your technique by undertaking the tutorial and exploring the materials on the British Hypertension Society (BHS) website.

Look at the make and last service date of the devices used in your workplace, and check them against the list of BHS-validated devices.

Consider the advantages and disadvantages of the different types of sphygmomanometer in use and think about how you might advise patients wishing to buy a device for use at home.

Download *Hypertension: Let's Do it Well*, a comprehensive learning pack for nurses available on the BHS website and suitable for individual or team updating. Work through the areas in which you wish to update your skills.

BOX 25.1   Measuring blood pressure: the auscultatory sounds[11]

Phase 1
The pressure reading at the first appearance of faint, repetitive, clear tapping sounds that gradually increase in intensity for at least two consecutive beats is the systolic blood pressure

Phase 2
A brief period may follow during which the sounds soften and acquire a swishing quality

Auscultatory gap
In some patients sounds may disappear altogether for a short time

Phase 3
The return of sharper sounds, which become crisper to regain or even exceed the intensity of phase 1 sounds (the clinical significance, if any, of phases 2 and 3 has not been established)

Phase 4
Distinct, abrupt, muffling sounds, which become soft and blowing in quality

Phase 5
The pressure reading when all sounds disappear completely is the diastolic pressure

---

Factors such as the service history of equipment, positioning of the patient, application and size of the cuff, too-rapid inflation/deflation of cuff, pressure on the stethoscope and impaired hearing are some of the factors that can influence readings.

Paired readings should be recorded, taken from each arm initially and the arm giving the higher reading noted for future reference. Standing blood pressure should be checked in elderly people and patients with diabetes to exclude postural hypotension.

The vibrations in the artery walls, heard via a stethoscope as the cuff is deflated, are known as the Korotkoff sounds. During deflation, the cuff pressure reaches a point where it is equal to the systolic pressure and blood starts to spurt through the artery. The sounds heard are divided into five phases (Box 25.1).

Continuous ambulatory blood pressure monitoring (CABM) may be useful in cases of 'white-coat' hypertension, where patients' blood pressure gives a high reading when it is measured by a healthcare worker, or when the blood pressure shows extreme variability or is resistant to treatment. The National Institute for Health and Clinical Excellence (NICE) does not recommend routine use of CABM in primary care as its value has not been adequately established.[12]

EFFECTS OF HYPERTENSION

Hypertension is a major risk factor for CHD, heart failure, stroke and renal failure. It has been described as a silent killer because serious damage can occur to the heart, brain and kidneys before any symptoms appear.

Hypertension promotes the formation of arteriosclerosis, pressure on the heart that can lead to CHD and heart failure and microvascular complications that can cause renal failure and retinal haemorrhage.

Treating hypertension also reduces morbidity and mortality from stroke. Even modest reductions in systolic and diastolic pressures can reduce stroke and CHD risks.[13]

DIAGNOSIS

Hypertension cannot be diagnosed from a single reading, as blood pressure may fluctuate widely during daily activities. NICE recommends that patients with persistent readings above 140/90 return for at least two more visits, when their blood pressure is assessed from two readings taken in the best conditions available.[12] Specialist intervention must be sought for patients with signs of secondary hypertension.[12]

Two new sets of guidelines were published in 2004 – from the BHS fourth working party and NICE. There are some differences in the guidelines relating to targets and the drug interventions. However, Campbell argues that there is only a minimal probability of benefit when target blood pressure or lipid measurements differences are small, and that the targets may be unachievable for many patients.[8]

MANAGEMENT

Lifestyle advice

Lifestyle interventions are indicated for all patients with hypertension, and as a primary prevention strategy. The practice nurse can support the patient to make these changes.

Health promotion should include advice on:

- smoking cessation, with access to counselling and treatment with nicotine replacement therapy and bupropion as indicated
- weight reduction to a body mass index of 20–25
- healthy eating, with at least five portions of fruit and vegetables a day, greater consumption of fish and foods containing polyunsaturated and monounsaturated fats, avoidance of foods high in saturated fat and caffeine-rich products (tea, coffee, cola drinks, chocolate bars and 'energy drinks') and reduced sodium intake
- limiting alcohol to 1–2 units a day

- regular aerobic exercise should be encouraged for 30 minutes a day, ideally on at least 5 days of the week
- relaxation therapy, which may be useful for some people.

Note that calcium, magnesium and potassium supplements are not indicated for blood pressure reduction.[12]

DRUG THERAPY

Many patients require drug therapy as well as lifestyle modification to lower blood pressure and prevent target-organ damage. Treatment should be offered to patients with persistent readings of 160/100 mmHg and over, and to those with a 10-year cardiovascular risk over 20% or a 10-year CHD risk over 15% and persistent blood pressure readings over 140/90 mmHg.[12]

The BHS and NICE guidelines differ in their approach to treatment. The BHS (Figure 25.1) differentiates between age groups and ethnic groups, and advocates an ABCD approach to managing therapy. The NICE guidelines (Figure 25.2) recommend starting from a universal point for every patient irrespective of age or ethnicity. The NICE summary suggests that monotherapy may be indicated in patients under the age of 55 years, and to consider starting with a beta

> **ACTIVITY**
>
> Using the British National Formulary and other resources such as Prodigy, review the broad categories of drug therapies indicated for the management of hypertension and relate the action of the drug to the physiological process it aims to modify.
>
> Check the contraindications and alternatives for sensitive patients.
>
> Find out which drugs are used commonly in your practice and review their action and use.
>
> Review the information leaflets on hypertension available on Prodigy, and consider how useful they might be as a resource for your patients.

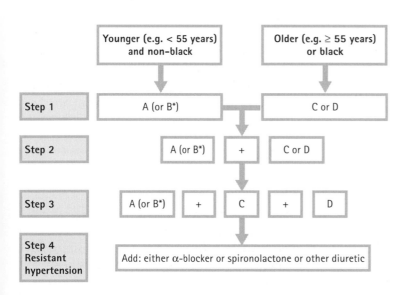

A ACE inhibitor or angiotensin receptor blocker
B Beta blocker
C Calcium channel blocker
D Diuretic (thiazide)

*Combination therapy involving B and D may induce more new-onset diabetes compared with other combination therapies

Adapted from the recommendations for combining blood pressure lowering drugs/ABCD rule

Figure 25.1   BHS recommendations for combining drugs.

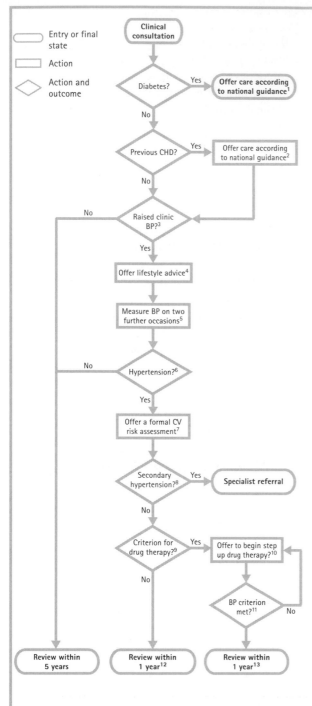

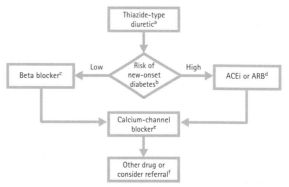

Entry or final state

Action

Action and outcome

3. Raised blood pressure (BP) > 140/90 mmHg (BP > 140/90 means either or both systolic and diastolic exceed threshold). Take a secondary confirmatory reading at the end of the consultation. Take a standing reading in patients with symptoms of postural hypotension.

4. Explain the potential consequences of raised BP. Promote healthy diet, regular exercise and smoking cessation.

5. Ask the patient to return for at least two subsequent clinics at monthly intervals, assessing BP under the best conditions available.

6. Hypertension: persistent raised BP > 140/90 mmHg at the last two visits.

7. Cardiovascular (CV) risk assessment may identify other modifiable risk factors and help explain the value of BP lowering and other treatment. Risk charts and calculators are less valid in patients with cardiovascular disease (CVD) or on treatment.

8. Refer patients with signs and symptoms of secondary hypertension to a specialist. Refer patients with malignant hypertension or suspected pheochromocytoma for immediate investigation.

9. Offer treatment for: (A) BP ≥ 160/100 mmHg; or
   (B) BP > 140/90 mmHg and 10-year coronary heart disease (CHD) risk ≥ 15%, CVD risk ≥ 20%, or existing CVD or target organ damage. Consider other treatments for raised cardiovascular risk, including lipid lowering and antiplatelet therapies.

10. As needed, add drugs in the following order:*

*If a drug is not tolerated discontinue and proceed to the next line of therapy. If a drug is tolerated but target BP is not achieved, add the next line of therapy. Drug cautions and contraindications are listed fully in the *British National Formulary*.

a. In young patients (under 55) whose BP may be managed on monotherapy, consider starting with a beta blocker.

b. Patients at high risk have a strong family history of type 2 diabetes, have impaired glucose tolerance (FPG ≥ 6.5 mmol/l), are clinically obese (BMI ≥ 30) or are of South-Asian or African-Carribean ethnic origin.

c. Beta blocker contraindications include asthma, chronic obstructive pulmonary disease and heart block.

d. Offer an angiotensin receptor blocker (ARB) if an angiotensin-converting enzyme inhibitor (ACEi) is not tolerated because of cough. Contraindications include known or suspected renovascular disease and pregnancy.

e. Only dihydropyridine calcium-channel blockers should be prescribed with a beta blocker. Contraindications include heart failure.

f. Consider offering a beta blocker or ACEi (if not yet used), another drug or specialist referral. A beta blocker and thiazide-type diuretic combination may become necessary in patients at high risk of developing diabetes if hypertension or CVD progress.

1. See the NICE guideline 'Management of Type 2 Diabetes: Management of Blood Pressure and Blood Lipids'.

2. See the NICE Guideline 'Prophylaxis for Patients who have Experienced a Myocardial Infarction: Drug Treatment, Cardiac Rehabilitation and Dietary Manipulation'.

11. BP ≥ 140/90 mmHg or further treatment is inappropriate or declined.

12. Check BP, reassess CV risk and discuss lifestyle.

13. Review patient care: medication, symptoms and lifestyle.

Figure 25.2   Management flowchart for hypertension. (*See footnote on page 189.)

blocker. The common theme of the two sets of guidance is that combination therapy should be used where necessary to lower blood pressure.

Other therapies

Blood pressure reduction is part of a cardiovascular risk reduction strategy. A cardiovascular risk assessment may indicate other interventions such as aspirin 75 mg/day or lipid-lowering therapy. It is important to recognise that the use of multiple drug treatments may raise concordance issues for patients. Where possible, drugs should be taken just once a day.[12]

ORGANISATION IN PRIMARY CARE

As it is a major risk factor for coronary heart disease and stroke, prevention and treatment of essential hypertension must be systematic and targeted. A practice register of patients with hypertension will facilitate regular contact and review through call–recall systems. All hypertensive patients must have their cardiovascular risk

> **LEARNING POINTS**
>
> - Two new sets of guidelines for hypertension were published in 2004
> - Hypertension is a major risk factor for CHD and stroke
> - All patients with hypertension require cardiovascular risk assessment
> - A multifactorial approach combining lifestyle modification and combination drug therapy may be necessary to reduce blood pressure
> - The GMS contract offers a potential 105 points for hypertension management

TABLE 25.2 How GMS quality points are earned in hypertension

Activity		Minimum target	Maximum target	Points
BP 1	The practice can produce a register of patients with established hypertension	NA	NA	9
BP 2	Percentage of patients with hypertension whose notes record smoking status at least once	25	90	10
BP 3	Percentage of patients with hypertension who smoke, whose notes contain a record that smoking cessation advice has been offered at least once	25	90	10
BP 4	Percentage of patients with hypertension in which there is a record of the blood pressure in the past 9 months	25	90	20
BP 5	Percentage of patients with hypertension in whom the most recent blood pressure (in the past 9 months) is 150/90 mmHg or less	25	70	56

*National Institute for Clinical Excellence (2004): 'Management flow chart for hypertension'. In: *Clinical Guideline 18: Hypertension – management of hypertension in adults in primary care.* London: National Institute for Clinical Excellence. Available from: http://www.nice.org.uk. Reproduced with permission of National Institute for Health and Clinical Excellence.

assessment recorded and updated. NICE recommends annual review, but practices are likely to need to see these patients more often.

Investigations include testing urine for protein, a blood sample for glucose, electrolytes, creatinine, total cholesterol and HDL cholesterol and a 12-lead ECG.[12] Other tests may be indicated where signs and symptoms suggest a secondary cause.

Management of patients with hypertension can earn a practice 105 quality points under the new GMS contract (Table 25.2).[14]

EVALUATION ACTIVITY

Reflect on your skills in interpreting the results of routine investigations for patients with hypertension. Are there areas in which you require further training or updating?

How does your team work together in the management of patients with hypertension? Are there any areas for improvement?

What has your practice achieved since the introduction of the new GMS contract?

REFERENCES

1. Laurent S. Guidelines from the British Hypertension Society [editorial]. BMJ 2004; 328: 593–594.
2. Wood D, Durrington P, Poulter N, et al. Joint British recommendations on prevention of coronary heart disease in clinical practice. Heart 1998; 80(Suppl 2): S1–S29.
3. Beevers DG, Churchill D (eds). Hypertension in Pregnancy, 3rd edn. London: Martin Dunitz, 1999, pp. 237–255.
4. British Hypertension Society. Guidelines for management of hypertension: report of the fourth working party of the British Hypertension Society – BHS IV. J Hum Hypertens 2004; 18: 139–185.
5. Department of Health. Saving Lives: Our Healthier Nation. London: The Stationery Office, 1999.
6. Department of Health. National Service Framework for Coronary Heart Disease. London: The Stationery Office, 2000.
7. Department of Health. Choosing Health: Making Healthier Choices Easier. London: The Stationery Office, 2004.
8. Campbell NC. Treating hypertension with guidelines in general practice (editorial). BMJ 2004; 329: 523–524.
9. Brady AJB. Introduction to hypertension. In: Brady AJB, Petrie JR (eds), New Perspectives on Hypertension. Basingstoke: Merit, 2003.
10. Hypertension: http://www.gpnotebook.co.uk
11. British Hypertension Society. Blood Pressure Measurement, 3rd edn. Available at: http://www.abdn.ac.uk/medical/bhs
12. NICE. Hypertension: Management of Hypertension in Adults in Primary Care. London: NICE, 2004.
13. Calhoun HM, Dong W, Poulter NR. Blood pressure screening, management and control in England: results from the Health of England Survey. J Hypertens 1998; 16: 747–752.
14. NHS Executive. The General Medical Services Contract. London: The Stationery Office, 2004.
15. Sharma S. Control of arterial blood pressure 1992; issue 1: article 5. Accepted 24/1/05. Available at: http://www.nda.ox.ac.uk/wfsa/html/u01/u01_008.htm

Section 4

Finding useful information

Chapter 26

Recognising the need for information

Debbie Fisher, Liz Fairclough and Maurice Wakeham

LEARNING OBJECTIVES

After reading this chapter you will be able to:

- define 'information' and identify some common key characteristics associated with the term
- describe a government information strategy that seeks to address the information needs of four distinct groups within the NHS: patients, healthcare professionals, managers and planners, and the public
- discuss research into the information needs of nurses

'Information' is often equated with 'knowledge', but both terms are defined and used inconsistently, so the complex relationship between the two remains confused. In this chapter we focus on how information affects and reflects knowledge and understanding.

It has been suggested that definitions of the word 'information' fall into one of three categories each of which is associated with 'knowledge' in a particular way (Box 26.1).[1] The three types of

---

ACTIVITY

What does the word 'information' mean to you?

Jot down your associations and examples to refer back to later in this chapter.

BOX 26.1   Definitions of 'information'

The many definitions of the word 'information' fall into three knowledge-related categories:

- **Learning**: information adds to and develops knowledge (information supplies and supports knowledge)
- **Uncertainty**: information reduces uncertainty (information is useful knowledge)
- **Expression**: knowledge communicated concerning some fact, subject or event (information is created by knowledge)

---

definitions may appear to conflict. However, key characteristics have been identified by researchers who have considered each type in the broad context of human knowledge:[1]

- *Uncertainty.* Information often reduces uncertainty about events in the real world, and this is often a primary motivation behind acquiring it.[1]
- *Knowledge.* Information affects our state of knowledge regarding something.
- *Ambiguity.* Information is always potentially ambiguous. We are required to interpret it within a context to identify precise meaning.
- *Indeterminacy.* A person who records (or sends) information has no absolute guarantee of (a) who exactly is going to receive it, and (b) how they are going to interpret it.
- *Redundancy.* The communication of information always has an element of redundancy (i.e. non-essential information), primarily to resolve problems of ambiguity and indeterminacy.
- *System dependency.* Messages must be carried by

ACTIVITY

Referring back to the notes you made in the last activity, can you recognise the three types of definitions and/or some of the key characteristics of the word 'information'?

---

a medium. People have to learn how to use this medium – to get the most out of the message.

If you were to associate, say, a bus timetable with 'information', you would see that the timetable could be said to:

- supply and support knowledge
- reduce uncertainty
- communicate facts.

The information contained within a bus timetable may:

- reduce uncertainty about the times when the bus may arrive at a bus stop
- allow you to plan your activities around the availability of transport
- not always be accurate – certain buses may not run or local problems may cause delays on the day
- confuse some people
- be too detailed
- be hard to read.

An individual's information needs will vary according to context and his or her role. In your personal life, knowing when a bus is due on a particular day is useful, but may not be essential information. In your professional role, your information needs are critically linked to providing care and developing professional knowledge and competence.

INFORMATION FOR HEALTH

The Government's view is that 'Better care for patients, and improved health for everyone, depend on the availability of good information, accessible when and where it is needed'.[2] The strategy document *Information for Health* outlines the Government's plans to:

> *Ensure that NHS clinicians and managers have the information needed to support the core purpose of the NHS, in caring for individuals and improving public health.*[2]

This strategy aims to meet the information needs of four distinct groups: patients, healthcare professionals, managers and planners, and the public.

Patients

Patients need information about:

- conditions
- treatments
- outcomes
- how to access health and social care services.

Healthcare professionals

Healthcare professionals need:

- fast, reliable and accurate information about individual patients in their care
- fast, easy access to local and national knowledge bases that support the direct care of patients and clinical management decision making
- access to information, to support them in the evaluation of the care they give, to underpin clinical governance, planning and research, and to help with their continuing professional development.

Managers and planners

Managers and planners need good quality information to help them target and use the resources deployed in the NHS, and to improve the quality of life of patients and local communities.

The public

The public need:

- convenient, accurate, up-to-date information about healthy living
- information about how the NHS is performing in the delivery of health care services (efficiency and outcomes)

- information to enable them to influence local service development, as well as local and national policy
- information to support self-treatment and care, where it is appropriate, so they know when to seek professional help and when and where to obtain it (e.g. from NHS Direct).

Person-centred approach to information

This 'person-centred' approach to information (to meet the needs of individuals) differs from previous strategies that have focused on the needs of the service – i.e. those of managers and planners.

ACTIVITY

In your professional role, when did you last seek information?

What precipitated this information need?

Make a note of this event and other examples of information needs that might arise in a practice context.

In the activity you may have referred to a need to:

- respond to a query from a patient/client/carer/relative/colleague
- find out more about a particular procedure or treatment
- contribute to the development of clinical guidelines or protocol
- implement research findings effectively
- prepare for an assignment, presentation or teaching session
- update your professional knowledge.

DEFINING AN INFORMATION NEED

Several research studies have been conducted to analyse the information needs of nurses and midwives. Some of the earlier studies referred to below were conducted when access to electronic sources may have been limited. Accessing relevant information may be easier now that information services are more developed. However, the findings still offer insights into the needs of nurses and midwives, and some of the problems they experience.

Personal interest

A study of nurses' information-seeking behaviour – carried out in 1991 by Anglia Polytechnic (now Anglia Ruskin University) in five local health districts – found that information was most likely to be required in relation to patient care or for personal interest or updating.[3]

The 'personal interest' category could include a whole range of reasons, which might also pertain to other categories, as the authors comment:

It is in the individual's interest to take an interest – to know about patients' problems and care needs, to be well informed about one's specialism, to be alert to current research, to be aware of job opportunities or possibilities for self development.

A study of the information needs of qualified nurses in the Bloomsbury Health Authority found that the most common reasons for seeking information were, first, to address clinical needs and, second, to address teaching and administrative needs.[4]

A more recent survey of health professionals' needs across the NHS found that the most often cited needs for information are: research, keeping up to date, education, continuing professional development and patient care.[5]

Professional concerns

A research project called EVINCE (Establishing the Value of Information to Nursing Continuing Education) was set up to examine the impact of information on the clinical knowledge and practice of nurses, midwives and health visitors. The study found that practitioners need information for the following reasons:[6]

- personal – updating knowledge/information, research, coursework
- patient care – specific drug or therapy, administration, rare condition or specific problem, and audit/standards/guidelines
- teaching – staff/students/colleagues and patient education
- publication
- research.

What has proved more difficult to be precise about is the influence on information needs of specific professional roles. The tendency for nurses, midwives and health visitors to be treated as homogeneous groups when discussing information requirements has been criticised, and a call made for those providing information services to recognise distinctions between, for example:[7]

A health visitor who has to give instantaneous responses to client needs in the community, a newly qualified staff nurse in an acute hospital just trying to survive the day, a midwife meeting the needs of a healthy mother, or a clinical nurse specialist functioning at an advanced practice level.

All of the above studies have tried to identify differences in information needs associated with specific professional roles; others have indicated differences in the pattern of information needs and use of midwives.[4, 8, 9] The EVINCE study attempted to make distinctions between groupings – such as acute and community staff and staff nurses and midwives – but the differences were not statistically significant.[5]

It has been suggested that differences in information need and use might be more distinct at an individual, rather than a group, level and that subjective assessments of the value of information may be more dependent on an individual's:[11]

- interest in continuing education than on the role implied by his or her job title
- level of practice, which can be used as an indicator of information need and use.

ACTIVITY

Look back at your response to the last activity.

To what extent are your information needs associated with your role?

Do you have information needs that extend beyond the boundaries of your job description?

Respondents to the EVINCE survey often had several purposes in mind for the information they sought. It appeared that their information needs were less specific than those of doctors (when the results were compared with a similar study looking at doctors' information needs and use). This might be related to the holistic nature of nursing and midwifery care, and the considerable and ongoing changes in care provision.[11]

Furthermore, changes in pre- and post-registration education mean that, in addition to the primary tasks associated with the provision of care, nurses and midwives may have other responsibilities – e.g. to act as mentors or supervisors – in addition to being students on post-registration courses.

Information gathered for one purpose may also be useful for others. A patient's enquiry about the purpose of pre-operative fasting, for example, may lead you to check out the latest research, which you then use to advise other patients and to form the basis of a teaching session for students or healthcare assistants.

CONCLUSION

There are many different types of information that you can draw upon to meet many different

---

EVALUATION ACTIVITY

Think about your information need examples.

How did you use the information you sought?

Can you identify any other opportunities for making further use of the information?

LEARNING POINTS

- Information affects and reflects knowledge and understanding
- Although definitions of 'information' may vary, and sometimes conflict, certain key common characteristics associated with the term can be identified: information reduces uncertainty, affects our state of knowledge, is always potentially ambiguous, may be indeterminate, usually contains redundant elements, and is dependent on the system used to convey it
- The information strategy for the NHS adopts a 'person-centred' approach to ensure that good quality information is available – when and where it is needed – to patients, healthcare professionals, managers and planners, and the public
- Research undertaken to analyse the information needs of nurses and midwives confirms the view that practitioners need:
  - fast, reliable and accurate information about individual patients/clients in their care
  - fast, easy access to local and national knowledge bases that support the direct care of patients/clients and clinical management decision making
  - access to information to support them in the evaluation of the care they give, underpinning clinical governance, planning and research and helping with their continuing professional development

types of information need. Your information needs will vary according to context and role, but information literacy is key to maintaining and developing your professional knowledge and competence. Once you have identified an information need, your next task will be to identify appropriate sources to bridge the information gap. In Chapter 27 we will look at different types of information, and the different formats in which they appear.

REFERENCES

1. Badenoch D, Reid C, Burton P, Gibb F, Oppenheim C. The value of information. In: Feeney M, Grieves M (eds), The Value and Impact of Information. East Grinstead: Bowker-Saur, 1994.
2. NHS Executive. Information for Health: An Information Strategy for the Modern NHS 1998–2005: A National Strategy for Local Implementation. London: NHS Executive, 1998.
3. Wakeham M, Houghton J, Beard S. The Information Needs and Information Seeking Behaviour of Nurses. British Library R&D Report 6078. London: British Library Board, 1992.
4. Williamson J. Information needs of qualified nurses in Bloomsbury Health Authority. Unpublished MPhil thesis, University College London, 1990.
5. Lindsay D, ward S, Winterman V. NHS Staff User Survey. London: TFPL Ltd, 2005.
6. Urquhart C, Davies R. EVINCE: the value of information in developing nursing knowledge and competence. Health Libraries Rev 1997; 14(2): 61–72.
7. Yeoh J. Editorial. Health Libraries Rev 1997; 14(2): 57–59.
8. Levine K. An assessment of the information needs of midwives and related health professionals and the extent to which current provision satisfied these needs. Unpublished MSc dissertation, University of Wales, Aberystwyth, 1993.
9. Bawden D, Robinson K. Information behaviour in nursing specialities: a case study of midwifery. J Inf Sci 1997; 23(6): 407–421.
10. Davies R, Urquhart CJ. EVINCE: Establishing the value of information to nursing continuing education. Report of the EVINCE Project. British Library Research and Innovation Centre Report 44. London: British Library, 1997.
11. Urquhart C. Personal knowledge: a clinical perspective from the VALUE and EVINCE projects in health library and information services. J Documentation 1998; 54(4): 420–442.

FURTHER INFORMATION

An online index with abstracts of all theses accepted for higher degrees by the Universities of Great Britain and Ireland is available. http://www.theses.com

Bandolier: a print and internet journal about evidence-based healthcare that provides advice for healthcare professionals about particular treatments. http://www.jr2.ox.ac.uk/bandolier

Cochrane Collaboration: an international not-for-profit organisation, providing up-to-date information about the effects of health care. It reviews healthcare interventions and promotes clinical trials and other studies. http://www.cochrane.org

National Electronic Library for Health (NeLH): provides information and access to virtual libraries. It facilitates discussion, collaboration and communication within the UK academic community and beyond. http://www.nelh.nhs.uk

Netting the Evidence: an introduction to researching evidence-based practice on the internet that aims to provide access to useful learning resources. http://www.shef.ac.uk/scharr/ir/netting

Nursing Midwifery and Allied Health Professions (NMAP): a gateway to internet resources aimed at students, researchers, academics and practitioners. http://www.nmap.ac.uk

Chapter 27

Addressing the information gap

Debbie Fisher, Liz Fairclough and Maurice Wakeham

LEARNING OBJECTIVES

After reading this chapter you will be able to:

- list a range of different information sources
- differentiate between primary and secondary sources
- discuss the role of systematic reviews and clinical guidelines as sources of information
- identify electronic sources of information

The nature of an individual's need for information and the context in which it arises will influence how the information is sought. In this chapter we focus on where you can go to obtain the information you need.

A major survey was carried out by the Royal College of Nursing (RCN) in 2004 of the information needs of nurses.[1] It was found that 43% of NHS nurses thought they used the library regularly and 60% felt thay had easy access to a library when they needed it. There was evidence that many nurses did not use or were not aware of the range of resources available to them on the internet, and over half thought they would benefit from instruction in information searching. As with other studies, visits to the library were predominantly for course-related or academic reasons. Students and others on formal courses tend to be aware of and use the wider range of resources available.[2, 3]

You may not find it easy to get to libraries or to find the time to use them, and the stock at accessible libraries may not be appropriate for your needs or specialty. Some of you may lack skills in using computers or are perhaps uncertain about how best to use libraries, or both – many studies have found that participants lack confidence and ability in information retrieval.[4, 5]

IDENTIFYING APPROPRIATE RESOURCES

Information is available from many different sources and in many different formats (Figure 27.1).

The EVINCE project, funded by the British Library Research and Innovation Centre, examined the impact of library and information services for nurses, midwives and health visitors on the competence and practice of those professionals. Its findings confirmed those of similar studies – demonstrating that practitioners rely on verbal sources as much as written sources, and want easily accessible and digestible information for patient/client care.[6]

Other researchers have found that nurses most often asked colleagues for information on patient care and the second choice was a practice-based resource.[5] Personal journal collections also proved popular.

As nursing is a practice-based profession, it may be considered reasonable for nurses to call first upon their colleagues for information. However, under their Code of Professional Conduct nurses are personally accountable for their practice and must maintain and improve their professional knowledge and competence.[7] Professional accountability rests on an individual's commitment to keep up to date with practice develop-

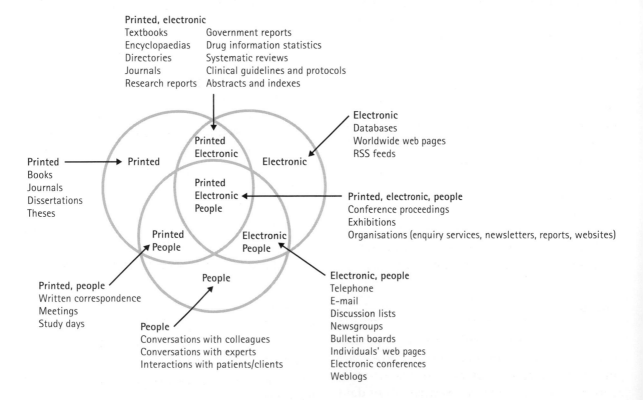

Figure 27.1   Key information sources: showing the impact of electronic developments.

ments and to provide a properly reasoned account of his or her actions. The shift towards evidence-based practice reinforces the need for nurses to develop their information skills to access the full range of available sources. Conventionally, these are divided into primary and secondary sources.

PRIMARY AND SECONDARY INFORMATION SOURCES

It is important to recognise the difference between primary and secondary sources of information. A primary source is an account of work carried out by the writer – e.g. a research report, an article, or a book. A secondary source describes work carried out by others – e.g. a literature review or bibliographic database.

Secondary sources provide useful overviews on subjects, commenting on and interpreting primary sources. However, if you wished to use information gathered from them for any particular purpose you would need to consult the primary sources (original work) referred to. It is not sufficient to rely on the accounts of others, be they verbal or in written form, because their interpretation may be faulty or biased. Nevertheless, secondary sources, such as bibliographic databases, systematic reviews and clinical guidelines, are vital elements of any information search.

Journals

Journals are a key source of information, particularly for research findings. Because they are published at regular intervals, journals generally contain information that is relatively up to date. Some, such as the *Journal of Advanced Nursing*,

give the date when an article was accepted for publication so that readers can assess the currency of its findings.

Nurses read journals 'to keep up to date with professional issues and trends, to keep up to date with current research, to find out more about clinical techniques'.[8]

In addition to the general nursing titles there are many journals that relate to specific areas of practice. In 1995, 40% of UK nursing journals had been established in the previous 5 years.[9] By 2000, CINAHL (Cumulative Index to Nursing and Allied Health Literature, a comprehensive bibliographic database for nursing titles) indexed 1,200 journals, compared with only 35 in 1961.

Journals can be categorised as:

- 'Primary' (academic), with content that is scholarly and research based – e.g. *Journal of Advanced Nursing*, *Nursing Research* and *International Journal of Nursing Studies*.
- 'Secondary' (professional), with content focusing on news items, practice issues, personal accounts, etc. – e.g. *Nursing Times*, *British Journal of Nursing* and *Practice Nurse*.

Electronic journals

Many journals are now available both on the worldwide web (see Further Information) and in print. This development has had a considerable impact on how journals are accessed and used. A subscription to a journal may allow you access to both forms. Some titles – e.g. the *Online Journal of Issues in Nursing* (http://www.nursingworld.org/ojin) – are freely available on the web with access to the current issue and archives.

In addition to bibliographic databases, libraries also offer electronic access to journals by subscribing to full-text services. These may be offered by individual publishers (e.g. ScienceDirect has more than 1000 full-text journals published by Elsevier Science) or groups of publishers (e.g. Ingenta contains full-text journals from more than 150 publishers). These full-text services act as databases, so you can search for information across the titles available.

Bibliographic databases can be linked to the full text of journal articles. Much will depend on what services individual libraries subscribe to (access to the electronic version of some journals is dependent upon the library also subscribing to the print version), so the content of some full-text services (such as Ingenta) may vary from library to library.

Remote access may be available – e.g. Royal College of Nursing members can register to access remotely some electronic journals the library subscribes to – or you may need to attend the institution to access full-text services.

The current situation is complex, but the potential is great. Remember, when you are browsing printed journals on the shelf in a library, that there may be many more available in electronic form.

Research reports

Research is published in a variety of formats, not just as articles in academic journals. Some studies are published in book form – e.g. some volumes of the Royal College of Nursing's Research Classics series have been reprinted several times since the 1970s.[10]

Organisations often publish research they have commissioned – e.g. the former Health Education Authority or the Mental Health Foundation.[11,12] The National Children's Bureau publishes authoritative summaries of research in its Highlight series. The Joseph Rowntree Foundation, which supports an extensive programme of research in social policy and social care, publishes summaries of research conclusions in a series called Findings, which is available in print and online.

Systematic reviews

Systematic reviews have a key role in supporting evidence-based practice. Although a secondary source they make it easier to find certain types of research to support or develop practice. The reviewers use systematic and explicit methods to:

- identify, select, and critically appraise available research on a subject
- collect and analyse data from studies that are included in the review
- analyse and summarise the results of the included studies.

Conclusions are based on a synthesis of studies that meet pre-set quality criteria.[13]

Reviewers use databases but also scan key journals in case any articles have been omitted or incorrectly indexed. They also contact individuals for details of research undertaken but not formally published. Systematic reviews are, therefore, more comprehensive and rigorous in approach than conventional literature reviews and offer a good guide to research in a particular field.[14]

The Cochrane Collaboration is an international collaboration committed to preparing, maintaining and disseminating systematic reviews of the effects of healthcare.[15] It produces the Cochrane Library, which includes the Cochrane Database of Systematic Reviews (containing approximately 3000 complete reviews and protocols) and the

Database of Abstracts of Reviews of Effects (DARE) (containing around 2000 abstracts of quality-assessed systematic reviews). DARE is an initiative of the Centre for Reviews and Dissemination, based at York University, which seeks to identify high-quality systematic reviews that have been published in journals and elsewhere.

Clinical guidelines

Clinical guidelines are developed, using information derived from systematic reviews or recommendations from primary research, to help practitioners to provide efficient and effective care.[16] Guideline development, whether at local, regional or national level, relies on multidisciplinary participation, although to date medical views have tended to predominate.[17] The National Institute for Health and Clinical Excellence (NICE) has a key role in coordinating the development and dissemination of clinical guidelines,[18] and further work is needed to establish how nurses and midwives could make more use of clinical guidelines in practice.[19]

The internet and the worldwide web

The internet is an international network of computers storing millions of pages of information. These pages are written in a programming language called hypertext mark-up language (html) that enables links to be made between them. The worldwide web (www) is the name given to these linked-up pages.

A commonly quoted description of the internet compares it to a library in shambles:

> *Information is organised on the internet as though you took all the books from a library, dumped them in a room and turned the light off.*[20]

The internet does, however, allow anyone with the appropriate technology to access much valu-able, and sometimes unique, information. The internet is, therefore, just another information source – albeit a vast and, in part, a chaotic one.

With access to the internet, you can:

- join 'virtual communities' to find out and exchange information, and benefit from the views of experts
- subscribe to email lists to receive selected information
- subscribe to newsgroups to read up-to-date news on a given subject.

There are bulletin boards, chat rooms, discussion forums and weblogs. You can observe (as a 'lurker') or subscribe and join in.

Most major organisations have their own intranets that use the same technology as the internet, but protect sensitive information by limiting access to staff (e.g. NHSnet for NHS staff).

IT developments, particularly the internet, have fundamentally changed how information is communicated and disseminated. The restrictions of time, place and space no longer apply in the same way.

CONCLUSION

You can address 'information gaps' by consulting a variety of primary and secondary sources, which may be available in verbal, written or electronic form. For information needs that arise in the context of practice you may refer, in the first

---

EVALUATION ACTIVITY

Consider a practice issue of interest to you.

Refer to Figure 27.1 and list the sources of information you would seek out to improve your knowledge of it.

Identify and distinguish between the primary and secondary sources, systematic reviews and practice-based evidence.

instance, to a colleague or to other secondary sources, such as relevant databases or literature reviews.

For more detailed information, you would need to consult a primary source (research reports, articles or books), particularly if you wanted to use the information gathered to inform clinical decision-making. In this instance, you cannot rely on the accounts of others (secondary sources), because their interpretations may be faulty or biased. One exception is, perhaps, the systematic review, which can offer a reliable account of research that has been undertaken in a particular field.

LEARNING POINTS

- We tend to rely on informal methods of information seeking, such as asking a colleague or referring to a practice-based resource
- We often cite a lack of confidence in our information retrieval skills as a reason for not using library and information services
- The internet, worldwide web and organisations' intranets are increasingly important sources of information
- The rise of evidence-based practice requires individual practitioners to develop information-gathering skills and to keep them up to date

---

REFERENCES

1. Bertulis R, Lord J, Keys J. Report of Key Findings of RCN's Survey of the Information Needs of Nurses, Health Care Assistants, Midwives and Health Visitors. London: Royal College of Nursing, 2005..
2. Bawden D, Robinson K. Information behaviour in nursing specialities: a case study of midwifery. J Inf Sci 1997; 23: 407–421.
3. Dee C, Stanley E. Information-seeking behaviour of nursing students and clinical nurses: implications for health sciences librarians. J Med Libraries Assoc 2005; 93(2).
4. Urquhart C, Crane S. Nurses' information-seeking skills and perceptions of information sources: assessment using vignettes. J Inf Sci 1994; 20: 237–246.
5. Wakeham M, Houghton J, Beard S. The Information Needs and Information Seeking Behaviour of Nurses. British Library R&D Report 6078. London: The British Library Board, 1992.
6. Urquhart C, Davies R. EVINCE: the value of information in developing nursing knowledge and competence. Health Libraries Rev 1997; 14: 61–72.
7. Nursing and Midwifery Council. Code of Professional Conduct, 2002. Available at: http://www.nmc-uk.org/nmc/main/publications/codeOfProfessionalConduct.pdf
8. Haig P. Nursing journals: are nurses using them? Nurs Stand 1993; 8(1): 22–25.
9. Stodulski AH. RCN Study of UK Nursing Journals. London: Royal College of Nursing Library & Information Service, 1995.
10. Hayward J, Boore JRP. Information: A Prescription Against Pain and Prescription for Recovery. RCN Research Classics. Harrow: Scutari Press, 1994.
11. Arthur S, Finch H. Physical Activity in our Lives: Qualitative Research Among Disabled People. London: Health Education Authority, 1999.
12. Mental Health Foundation. Knowing Our Own Minds: A Survey of How People in Emotional Distress Take Control of their Lives. London: Mental Health Foundation, 1997.
13. Crombie IK, McQuay HJ. The systematic review: a good guide rather than a guarantee. Pain 1998; 76(1/2): 1–2.
14. Nelson EA. The value of systematic reviews in research. Prof Nurse 1998; 14: 24–28.
15. Cochrane Collaboration. The Cochrane Collaboration: Preparing, Maintaining and Promoting Accessibility of Systematic Reviews of Effectiveness of Healthcare Intervention. Available at: http://www.cochrane.org
16. Paisley S. Filtering and evaluating the knowledge base. In: Booth A, Walton G (eds), Managing Knowledge in Health Services. London: Library Association, 2000, pp. 251–267.
17. Thomas L. Clinical practice guidelines. Evidence-based Nurs 1999; 2(2): 38–39.
18. Roberts R. Information for Evidence-Based Care. Oxford: Radcliffe Medical Press, 1999.
19. Thomas LH, McColl E, Cullum N, Rosseau N, Soutter J. Clinical guidelines in nursing, midwifery and the therapies: a systematic review. J Adv Nurs 1999; 30: 40–50.
20. Frankenburg B, former CEO of Novell, cited by Poulos B in: The Internet: the Challenges of Moving from Transport to Content – Where are the Opportunities? Speech delivered at the Canadian Resale IXC Industry Congress, 6 February 1996. Available at: http://www.telesat.ca/eng/speeches96–1.htm

FURTHER INFORMATION

Database of Abstracts of Reviews of Effectiveness (DARE): systematic reviews identified by searching bibliographic databases, medical journals and grey literature (i.e. reports, dissertations, product information, budgetary data and research findings made available by organisations other than publishers). DARE is also in the Cochrane Library, but this version contains more information. http://www.york.ac.uk/inst/crd/index.htm

MEDLINE: One of the most comprehensive indexes to medical literature, covering more than 4000 journals from 1966 onwards. Also includes the International Nursing Index. One MEDLINE site is PubMed: http://www.ncbi.nlm.nih.gov/PubMed

NHS Economic Evaluation Database (NHSEED): structured abstracts of economic evaluations of healthcare interventions. Includes cost–benefit analyses, cost–utility analyses and cost-effectiveness analyses of treatments or care alternatives, selected from a variety of sources against strict criteria. NHSEED is included in the Cochrane Library database, but is also available at: http://www.york.ac.uk/inst/crd/nhsdfaq.htm

Chapter 28

Strategies for locating information

Debbie Fisher, Liz Fairclough and Maurice Wakeham

LEARNING OBJECTIVES

After reading this chapter you will be able to:

- articulate your information need
- outline the steps involved in finding information
- develop a systematic method for locating the information you require
- understand how bibliographic databases are constructed and how they operate

Consider for a moment what you understand by the term 'systematic search'. Think of a search for information that you have recently undertaken: would a more systematic approach have helped, and in what way?

A SYSTEMATIC APPROACH

Nurses must be able to conduct a systematic search for information if they are 'to question their practice, management or education in a structured and meaningful way'.[1] This chapter introduces a nine-step model to help you to locate information systematically. The key steps have been presented in a particular order, but the search process is often iterative. Indeed, working through the cycles within the process is part of the skill of searching – seek and you will discover – so at any stage you may need to modify your search in the light of new information.

Systematic searching: key steps

All searches are likely to include some of the key steps outlined in Box 28.1. The level of enquiry will vary according to the purpose of the search and the time available, but the more you practise using this systematic approach, the better able you will be to construct search strategies appropriate to differing information needs.

DEFINING YOUR INFORMATION NEED

It is worth first spending some time thinking about the nature of your information need, because it will help you to determine the scope and extent of your search. Break the question down into its constituent parts, so that you understand exactly what you need to find out.

Let us say, as an example, that you have been asked to present a short paper to colleagues as part of an in-house programme of continuing

---

BOX 28.1   The key steps in a systematic search for information

- Define your information need
- Identify key words and concepts
- Set parameters for the search
- Identify types of information/appropriate sources
- Plan how to obtain/access these sources
- Carry out your search and record the results
- Evaluate your search results, and prioritise what you will follow up
- Locate items
- Evaluate items and the information you have found

---

professional development. Your allotted topic is 'Theories of pain: a review and update'.

Defining broad terms

Having articulated your information need, you will need to identify broad terms to describe the different parts of the question you are investigating – in this case 'pain' and 'theory'.

Thinking around the question

Think around the question: what type of issues might you need to explore? Make some preliminary, informal enquiries: consult reference texts or discuss your question with colleagues, or seek advice from people you know with expertise in the area. Keep notes about what is said. In the present example, issues you identify relating to 'theories of pain' might include:

- What counts as a 'theory'?
- When were the first theories of pain developed, and by whom?
- Is pain just one thing? Is emotional pain the same as physical pain?
- Why do we get pain?
- Is there one current dominant theory of pain or several?
- How have theories of pain developed over time?
- How can understanding theories of pain help when working with patients in pain?

KEY WORDS AND CONCEPTS

If, as you collect information and ideas about your question, you jot down in any order all the words you associate with it, you can then make a spray diagram (Figure 28.1).[2] Spray diagrams help you to identify relationships between subjects, and the process of rearranging the information you are gathering promotes learning and understanding.

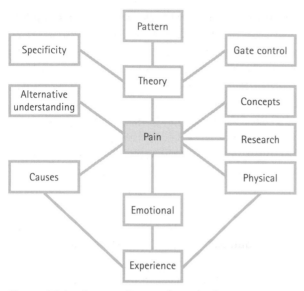

Figure 28.1   A spray diagram for pain theory.

At this stage in your search you may not be sure whether you wish to focus on specific or general issues. In our example, you could focus on a specific aspect of the subject of pain (e.g. how anxiety might impact on the experience of pain), or you could deal with the subject in broader terms and address the experience of pain as one part of your presentation.

ACTIVITY

Identify an area of your own practice that you would like to know more about.

Make a spray diagram to help.

Think around the question and make preliminary enquiries.

Identify the key words and concepts pertaining to your question/subject area.

The key words and concepts identified in the activity above are what you will need to guide your search for information. The key words will become your 'search terms' when you delve into indexes or 'the literature' catalogued by electronic databases such as the British Nursing Index (BNI),

Cumulative Index to Nursing and Allied Health Literature (CINAHL) and MEDLINE (see below).

It is usually a good idea to make your search terms as specific as possible. If you choose broad terms, you could be overwhelmed by the results of your search, and may need to narrow them down, although if they are too specific you might not get all the information you need. For example, using 'pain or theory' as a search term to interrogate a database is likely to result in too many hits. Using 'pain theory' or 'pain and theory' will reduce the number of hits.

Luckily, databases often include indexes and thesauri to help you select appropriate terms. For example, if you are specifically searching for information about cultural aspects of pain, the British Nursing Index uses 'pain ethnography' as a subject term. Bear in mind that different databases have different search interfaces – i.e. likely to vary in the way search screens are set up and information is presented.

SETTING SEARCH PARAMETERS

The extent of your search will be determined by the nature of your information need. Every search has an end and some searches are shorter than others. Setting the parameters of your search means setting limits to it. For example:

- How much time do you have?
- How many years back does your search need to go? Do key dates apply? (For example, you would not expect to find many references in databases to HIV before the mid- to late 1980s.)
- Do articles need to be in English? (Many databases provide records in English of material written in another language.)

IDENTIFYING APPROPRIATE SOURCES

For background information – facts and general principles – up-to-date textbooks are a good starting point. They also offer useful summaries of possibly complex topics or help to set them in context.

Databases

For most searches, journals are a key source of information. To pick out relevant articles you will need to use electronic 'bibliographic' databases such as the BNI, CINAHL and MEDLINE, which are available online via the web or on CD-ROMs.

Bibliographic databases usually cover a particular subject field and enable flexible and effective searching, usually across a wide range of journals over a number of years. The references they provide are citations of published studies (e.g. Shawe J, Ineichen B. Using a youth café to provide contraceptive services. *Primary Health Care* 2000; 10(5): 37–40) that usually incorporate an abstract or annotation summarising the content of the article, to inform your decision about whether to follow up that particular reference.

CINAHL is the most comprehensive database; it indexes more than 1,200 journals, with references to articles from 1982 onwards.[3] BNI's coverage is strictly that of nursing and midwifery from a UK standpoint. Some databases include types of literature other than journal articles; for example, CINAHL includes some books and dissertations (usually American). Material indexed by the BNI and not by CINAHL includes the *British Journal of General Practice*.

Increasingly, databases enable you to go beyond the abstracts and access the full text of some of the articles. What you will be able to access, and how, will depend to some extent on which of a wide range of full-text services your library, or employer, subscribes to and how these are combined.

The boundaries between what is primarily a bibliographic database and what is a full-text journal database are becoming increasingly blurred. A library is likely to have both types, and you may need to search all those that are appropriate to your information need. For example, you may be able to access some journals using Ingenta, but would perhaps need to refer to CINAHL to find out what might be available across a broader range of British and American nursing journals.

Some databases will be more appropriate than others, but there are no hard and fast rules. The relative merits of CINAHL and MEDLINE for nursing searches have been debated in terms of relevance and numbers of references.[4]

Accessibility of the articles found may also be a consideration. It is usually worth searching on several databases, depending on how comprehensive you want to be in your search and how much time you have. It can be interesting to see if different databases come up with similar or very different results. The former can help to confirm that you have tracked down the main sources, while the latter can help open up your search in other directions.

ACTIVITY
Identify how you would best use online databases to further the search for information on your chosen topic.

Distilled and consolidated sources

Secondary sources that can speed up a search have been described as 'sources of distilled and consolidated information'.[5] For example, the journals *Evidence-based Nursing* and *Evidence-based Mental Health* provide abstracts of high-quality research with an accompanying commentary.

Bandolier is a freely available online journal, developed specifically to support evidence-based practice. It distils information from reviews, randomised controlled trials and other quality studies, bringing the information together in a more comprehensible and accessible format.

WHAT IS BEST EVIDENCE?

If nursing practice is to be evidence based, the 'best evidence' must be sought. But what is 'best evidence'? Different information sources can be categorised according to the strength of evidence they provide in answer to particular types of question – a process sometimes referred to as establishing a 'hierarchy of evidence'.[6] The quality of evidence gathered in any search, however, will depend upon the question asked.

A commonly cited 'hierarchy of evidence' places research studies that use randomised controlled trials (RCTs) at the top of the hierarchy, and expert opinions or the opinions of 'respected authorities' at the bottom of the hierarchy.[6] RCTs are regarded as the gold standard of evidence, because they are considered the most rigorous and least biased type of study. The Cochrane Library contains a database of RCTs that provide the focus of many systematic reviews. Properly conducted RCTs provide important evidence for the effectiveness of interventions for all health professionals. However, there are concerns about the tendency to value RCTs in particular, and quantitative research in general, more highly than all other forms of research, including qualitative studies, and the impact that this might have on nursing practice; these concerns are expressed in the remark that 'evidence for nursing should reflect the different orientation of nursing practice and research'.[7]

A definition of what constitutes evidence-based practice in a given situation will be determined by three key elements:

- external best evidence
- clinical expertise and experience
- the individual patient's situation and preferences.

Some feel that too much reliance is placed upon external evidence. They argue that the findings of large-scale, quantitative research studies, for example, may not be readily applicable to the individualised, holistic care that is central to nursing.[8] It has also been suggested that anecdotal evidence has a place within the synthesis of clinical expertise and best evidence, and there have been calls for different approaches to research to take intuitive approaches and experience into account.[9]

CONCLUSION

In this chapter we have explored how to develop a systematic approach to the search for information. Although it has been presented as a staged process, in which each step relies on those

---

LEARNING POINTS

- The ability to conduct a systematic search for information is essential if nurses are to question their practice, management or education in a structured and meaningful way
- A systematic search for information is an iterative process
- Time spent at the outset of a search, thinking about the nature of your information need, will help you to determine its scope and extent
- When you have defined your information need, identify the key words and concepts associated with your enquiry – these will act as your search terms
- Set the parameters of your search. Every search has an end. The extent of your search will be determined by the nature of your information need
- You can consult a wide range of sources of information: books and journals, bibliographic and full-text databases, systematic reviews, etc. You need to match the most appropriate source(s) to your information need
- Some types of information are more highly valued than others, but 'best' evidence will depend on the content and context of the question being addressed

previously taken, searching for information is usually an iterative process. In the light of information gathered at any stage you may need to return to previous positions, to refocus your search. However, assuming that you have defined your information need, identified key words and concepts, set parameters for your search and identified the types of information/appropriate sources you wish to access, you will now be well placed to achieve the desired outcome.

EVALUATION ACTIVITY

Summarise how taking the steps described above have assisted you in refining the search for information on the topic you identified earlier.

REFERENCES

1. Benton DC, Cormack DFS. Searching the literature. In: Cormack DFS (ed.), The Research Process in Nursing, 4th edn. Edinburgh: Blackwell Science, 2000; pp. 89–102.
2. Buzan T, Buzan B. The Mind Map Book. London: BBC Consumer Publishing, 2003.
3. CINAHL. History: Then and Now, 2000. Available at: http://www.cinahl.com/about/ abt-history.htm
4. Brazier H, Begley CM. Selecting a database for literature searches in nursing: MEDLINE or CINAHL? J Adv Nurs 1996; 24: 868–875.
5. McKibbon KA, Marks S. Searching for the best evidence. Part 1: Where to look. Evidence-based Nurs 1998; 1(3): 68–70.
6. Muir Gray JA. Evidence-based Healthcare, 2nd edn. Edinburgh: Churchill Livingstone, 2001.
7. James T, Smith P. Implementing research: the practice. In: Mulhall A, le May A (eds), Nursing Research: Dissemination and Implementation. Edinburgh: Churchill Livingstone, 1999, pp. 177–204.
8. Urquhart C. Personal knowledge: a clinical perspective from the VALUE and EVINCE projects in health library and information services. J Documentation 1998; 54: 420–442.
9. McCutcheon H, Pincombe J. Intuition: an important tool in the practice of nursing. J Adv Nurs 2001; 35: 342–348.

Index